T0386701

THE LAST AND LONGEST MILE

FUMIHIKO TAKAYAMA

The Last and Longest Mile

Yohei Sasakawa's Struggle to Eliminate Leprosy

Translated by
Waku Miller

HURST & COMPANY, LONDON

First published in the United Kingdom in 2021 by
C. Hurst & Co. (Publishers) Ltd.,
41 Great Russell Street, London, WC1B 3PL

Distributed in the United States, Canada and Latin America by Oxford University
Press, 198 Madison Avenue, New York, NY 10016, United States of America.

A Cataloguing-in-Publication data record for this book
is available from the British Library.

ISBN: 9781787383401

www.hurstpublishers.com

CONTENTS

AUTHOR'S PREFACE TO THE ENGLISH EDITION

On the following pages are episodes from the fight to eradicate leprosy by Yohei Sasakawa and the organization that he leads, the Nippon Foundation. Leprosy and the unfounded discrimination that it occasions have blighted humankind throughout history. The episodes related here detail how Yohei has extended a helping hand to individuals afflicted by that blight.

Yohei has stridden for nearly half a century in the vanguard of the struggle to end the indescribable suffering caused by leprosy. His role in that struggle figures prominently in my biography of Yohei and his father, Ryoichi, *Shukumei no ko—Sasakawa ichizoku no shinwa* (Destiny's children—the Sasakawa family mythology) (Tokyo: Kodansha, 2014). The dual-biography format precluded, however, a proper treatment of the vast scope—chronological, geographical, cultural, and religious—of Yohei's crusade against leprosy. I have endeavored in this book to provide readers with a multifaceted portrayal of that crusade.

Tackling discrimination along with the disease

Let us note that Yohei's struggle against leprosy is more than a fight to eradicate the disease. It is also a campaign to eradicate the discrimination suffered by sufferers and recoverees and by their family members.

The World Health Organization (WHO) set the goal in 1991 of eliminating leprosy "as a public health problem" by 2000. It defined that goal as reducing leprosy's prevalence to less than 1 per 10,000 persons in every nation. Thanks to such determined spirits as Yohei, the struggle had largely attained the WHO's goal by the turn of the century. Medical science had developed an effective pharmaceutical regimen for curing leprosy by the 1980s, and making the medicine available worldwide, supported by funding from Yohei's Nippon Foundation, turned the tide against the disease.

Discrimination has proved more intractable than the physiological disease. Individuals who have contracted leprosy suffer social ostracism even after they have been cured. Any aftereffects of leprosy mark them in the eyes of the ignorant and prejudiced as unclean, as carriers of disease, even as subjects of divine wrath. Yohei has railed against such prejudice, making his case even face-to-face with presidents and ministers of health.

"Bringing leprosy under control," he argues, "is only part of the solution. This is a serious human rights issue. We need to accompany measures for bringing and keeping the disease under control with educational efforts aimed at eliminating discrimination. Bringing the disease under control and eliminating discrimination are like the two wheels of a motorcycle. Genuine progress depends on putting both wheels in place. Let us shape a world where discrimination against sufferers and former sufferers of leprosy and their family members is a thing of the past. Only then will we be able to say that we have fulfilled our mission."

The notion of leprosy as a divine punishment for untold sins has exercised a powerful hold on humanity for millennia. Those who would undo that hold encounter stubborn resistance in each nation in the form of cultural and religious prejudice. Even Yohei's most fervent supporters sometimes flash looks that betray doubts about his prospects for success.

Leprosy, though communicable, has never been as contagious as people have feared through the ages. And it is today entirely curable. Yet leprosy has engendered more prejudice, more discrimination than any other disease. That is presumably because of the severe and highly visible disfigurement that it wrought on victims before a cure became available and that it still wreaks if left untreated.

The persecution experienced by persons who have contracted leprosy and by their family members is remarkably similar across the nations of the world. Persons who contract the disease have frequently suffered expulsion from their homes and villages. Even uninfected family members of individuals who have contracted leprosy have been subject to such expulsion.

The biblical roots of prejudice

In Western cultures, attitudes and behaviors toward leprosy reflect the numerous disparaging references to the disease in the Bible, in both the New Testament and Old Testament. European nations carried that prejudice around the world in the Age of Discovery, starting in the 15th century. They colonized territory across Africa, Asia, and the Americas, destroying the religions of the local peoples, enslaving countless individuals, slaughtering countless others. A driving force in the European onslaught was Christian zeal, as documented in numerous histories of the era.

Prejudice against persons affected by leprosy, meanwhile, was part and parcel of Christianity on account of the biblical references. Yet those references reflect fundamental misunderstanding of the disease supposedly in question. In fact, the disease caused by *Mycobacterium leprae* and known as leprosy did not exist in the Middle East in biblical times. Hebrew-to-Greek translators rendered the Hebrew *tsara'at*, which refers to a broad range of skin conditions, as the Greek *lepra*. Subsequent translations of the Bible followed their lead in rendering the term as "leprosy" or "leper" in English and as equivalent terms in other languages.

Troubling enough is the mistranslation of *tsara'at*. Translators compounded the problem, meanwhile, with rhetorical flourishes that inserted "leprosy" or "leper" where *tsara'at* was absent in the Hebrew original. A notorious example is the Douay-Rheims Bible's rendering of Isaiah 53:1–5, which prophesizes Jesus's suffering on behalf of humanity:

> Who hath believed our report? and to whom is the arm of the Lord revealed? Despised, and the most abject of men, a man of sorrows, and acquainted with infirmity: and his look was as it were hidden and despised, whereupon we esteemed him not. Surely he hath borne our infirmities and carried our sorrows: and we have thought him as it were a leper, and as one struck by God and afflicted. But he was wounded for our iniquities, he was bruised for our sins: the chastisement of our peace was upon him, and by his bruises we are healed.

The Douay-Rheims Bible, published in 1582 (New Testament) and in 1609 and 1610 (Old Testament), is an English translation of a Latin translation from Greek and Hebrew sources by Jerome of Stridon (347–420), Saint Jerome. In the passage cited, Jerome has taken a leap of translation in associating the Hebrew *nagua* and *mukkay*—*percussum* and *humiliatum* in his Vulgate rendering and "struck" and "afflicted" in the Douay-Rheimes translation—with leprosy. He has emphasized that association by adding the phrase *quasi leprosum*—"as it were a leper" in the Douay-Rheimes translation. No text that corresponds to that phrase appears in either the Greek or Hebrew originals. And the translators of the King James, Revised Standard, and New International versions of the Bible have mercifully eschewed Jerome's inapt addition.

An unprecedented crusader

Semi-mythical figures of different religious traditions and historical figures in different nations have tended to persons afflicted by leprosy. Yohei is the first individual, however, who has worked so passionately and so effectively to end the prejudice and discrimination that the disease engenders. He has strived tirelessly to defang the horrific misconceptions that underlie the continuing persecution of innocent people.

Yohei's work to transform awareness and eliminate discrimination inherently entails criticizing policy and public administration in different nations. It has entailed, too, criticizing religions and religious figures that have resorted to discrimination against persons affected by leprosy in their evangelism.

Yohei's crusade is nothing less than an effort to undo a collective illusion that humankind has conjured over millennia. He is calling for a rethinking of basic precepts of civilization. This is a bold undertaking, overlapping the realm of the philosophical. "What is being human all about?" Yohei asks. "What is the meaning of life?"

I have appended to the chronicle of Yohei's travels on the following pages a historical overview of leprosy, including religious and national perspectives. The history of leprosy is a long, dark tale of how humankind has disseminated, sometimes knowingly, mistaken notions. It is a revelation of how religions have used that dissemination to exert a hold on minds.

Political power has mingled with religions' misleading thought. In 20th-century Japan, the government, in the name of ethnic cleansing, herded persons afflicted with leprosy into prison-like sanatoriums. Those individuals suffered a fate akin to being erased from society.

Southeast Asian nations colonized by Western powers were long the scene of forced isolation in leprosariums on islands. Similar facilities stood on the Hawaiian island of Molokai and the Greek island of Spinalonga. The overseers prohibited the residents, of course, from procreating. When residents somehow managed to bear children despite the prohibition, those offspring suffered the fate of lifelong confinement to their island. The idea was to isolate all persons who had contracted leprosy until the last one had perished. It was analogous to the Nazi thinking that underlaid the Holocaust. We can but shudder at the realization that two holocausts unfolded simultaneously in recent history.

History ought to be more than a hindsighted exercise in citing our forebears for their sins. We have a responsibility as members of society to come to terms with history. That means examining why the unspeakable occurred, why people behaved as they did. It also means bringing a humble and scientific approach to the task of identifying a better course for civilization in the years ahead.

AUTHOR'S PREFACE TO THE ENGLISH EDITION

We can regard the history of leprosy as the history of humankind, as the history of religion and of civilization. That is because it fairly throbs with the ineffable essence of human life. Standing alongside Yohei Sasakawa, I have beheld tableaus of hopelessness so bracing as to make me quiver and sometimes even quake. And I realized as I completed this work that Yohei's crusade is an eternal undertaking.

Fumihiko Takayama

AUTHOR'S PREFACE TO THE JAPANESE EDITION

This book offers a look at Nippon Foundation chairman Yohei Sasakawa engaged in his lifetime quest: working to eradicate leprosy and to eradicate prejudice against leprosy's victims. That quest has been a global undertaking, and I recount here episodes from our travels together to 20 nations from 2010 to 2016. Those travels took us to settings where I would never have set foot in the course of ordinary journeying: urban and remote leprosy colonies in India, tropical rainforests in Africa, jungle and desert in Brazil, the equatorial atolls of Kiribati.

People in the world's rich nations tend to regard leprosy as a thing of the past. Surprisingly few realize that leprosy continues to afflict numerous individuals around the world, especially where sanitation and nutrition are inadequate. Accompanying Yohei, I witnessed firsthand the reactions of people in Brazil and in Kiribati who had just received the diagnosis of leprosy. That included an entire family in Brazil. I'll never forget the profound sadness occasioned by the terrifying news.

Victims of leprosy have suffered social ostracism and other discrimination over the centuries. That is partly because the Judeo-Christian and Buddhist scriptures have misrepresented the disease as divine punishment for ostensible misdeeds. Discrimination has frequently inspired its victims to assert a separate but vigorous sense of community. Time and again, I have seen how victims of discrimination can muster familial ties of affection and mutual assistance. Neighborhoods of leprosy patients and former patients and their family members sometimes exhibit a closer-knit social fabric than is common in "ordinary" communities.

The symposium described in chapter 11 showcased the camaraderie and the generosity that animate the global community of persons affected by leprosy. Cohosting the symposium, which took place in the Vatican City, were the Nippon Foundation and the Holy See. On hand for the gathering were former patients and representatives of support organizations from around the world, as well as medical experts, religious figures, and other participants. Especially striking about the comments by the former patients was the lack of bitterness about their mistreatment and the sense of forgiveness toward their former tormenters.

While admiring the forgiving spirit displayed by discrimination's victims, let us be alert to the persistent specter of unfounded prejudice. Jesus might have healed sufferers of leprosy, but he didn't free them from discrimination. Gandhi and Mother Teresa offered leprosy sufferers solace but not liberation from discrimination. I have witnessed a miracle. I have seen a Japanese man parry the curse of discrimination against the victims of leprosy. And I am eager for readers to know that man.

Fumihiko Takayama

1

HEROISM AMID BEGGARY
MUMBAI AND PUNE

My travels with Yohei Sasakawa on his globe-trotting crusade against leprosy began in mid-December 2010. We took a direct flight on All Nippon Airways to Mumbai, in the state of Maharashtra on India's west coast. Over the next seven years, I would accompany Yohei on his leprosy-fighting travels to 20 nations.

India was an especially high priority for Yohei in fighting leprosy. The nation is home to some 12 million people who have or formerly had the disease—about 70% of the global total. That number is partly a reflection of India's massive population. With 1.26 billion people, India is the world's second most populous nation, after China. But the problem in India is primarily the result of severe and widespread poverty, which engenders conditions conducive to the disease. China has achieved a far lower incidence of leprosy, largely through greater progress in reducing malnutrition and in increasing access to sanitation services and medical care.

Complicating the task of health management in India is the nation's astonishing cultural and linguistic diversity. India has more than 2,000 ethnic groups. As for religion, about 80% of the people characterize themselves as Hindu, but Islam accounts for a double-digit share of the population, and India also has large communities of Christians, Sikhs, Buddhists, and Jains. The total number of living languages in the nation is somewhere between 300 and nearly 800, depending on what you classify as "dialects" or "languages." India's constitution designates Hindi and English as the official languages for conducting government business. It also grants official status to 21 other languages.

Another barrier to progress in improving health management in India is the ancient yet enduring Hindu system of castes. Discrimination based on caste persists despite a constitutional prohibition. It is especially onerous in the treatment of the members of the Dalit castes, at the bottom of the hierarchy. Caste is hereditary and fundamentally inescapable. Dalits' only exit from their caste-imposed fate is to leave the Hindu faith and take up a religion, such as Islam or Christianity, that rejects caste. That can entail, however, estrangement from their families, since religion is fundamental to family ties in India.

Hindu tradition restricts Dalits' vocational prospects to such work as slaughtering animals, producing leather goods, and cleaning up the human excrement that litters cityscapes nationwide. The Dalits' status as "untouchables" long prevented them from entering hospitals and clinics to receive medical care. It condemned those who contracted leprosy to a fate of physical deterioration and disfigurement.

Against all odds, India overcame the daunting obstacles cited here and achieved, miraculously, the benchmark prescribed by the World Health Organization (WHO) for eliminating leprosy as a public health problem: less than 1 active case per 10,000 population. The WHO put forth that benchmark in 1991. Evidence suggests that leprosy tends to decline naturally when its incidence declines below that level.

India attained the WHO benchmark in December 2005, and the government announced the accomplishment officially the following month. The nation's success in bringing leprosy under control ranks as a historic milestone in the fight against leprosy. Yohei expressed diffidence, however, about the achievement.

"This is a gratifying reward, to be sure, for years of striving to bring the disease under control, and it has reinforced confidence in our approach. It is also encouraging in that bringing the disease under control demonstrates real potential for eradicating it completely. We need to bear in mind, however, that the Indian government's announcement pertains to the nation as a whole. The rate of incidence is still above the benchmark in some states, and it remains above the benchmark in some districts in states that have attained the benchmark overall."

Yohei was keenly attentive to the troubling occurrence of large numbers of new cases each year in India: about 135,000 annually nationwide. He was equally attentive to the discrepancies among India's 29 states and seven union territories in progress in controlling leprosy. His data verified that the overall prevalence of leprosy in India was indeed below the WHO's elimination benchmark: 0.69 per 10,000 population at the time of our visit. It remained above the benchmark, however, in two states and in a union territory. Below the state and territory level, leprosy's prevalence was above the benchmark in 209 of India's approximately 650 administrative districts. More than half of the nation's states and union territories had one or more districts where the prevalence was above the benchmark.

A tearful grad student from Mumbai

India has some 1,000 leprosy sanatoriums and colonies. We headed directly for a large urban colony the morning after our arrival: the Sanjay Nagar leprosy colony, in the Borivali district of northwest Mumbai. This was the second visit to the colony for Yohei, who had been there previously in 2007.

Sanjay Nagar was a sprawling community, home to some 750 patients, former patients, and family members at the time of our visit. The colony dated as a refuge for society's outcasts from the 1940s. It originated on a forested site opposite a cremation ground. Three or four Dalit families had fled persecution and taken up residence there, and the wealthy landowner had permitted them to continue residing on her property. Other Dalits joined them over the years. Some of the residents were leprosy patients, and they developed a sense of camaraderie that became the foundation for the present colony.

Development had transformed the colony's setting profoundly over the past half century. A network of streets and roads had taken shape across the landscape, and condominiums and retail emporiums had sprung up among the venerable small shops along the larger thoroughfares on the colony's periphery. An overhead freeway passed nearby. The commercial spectrum was impressive. Among the establishments that happened to catch my eye around the colony were computer shops, dry cleaners, barbers, bicycle and motorcycle repair shops, carpenters, and cafés. All of the proprietors, we learned, were Dalits.

About 150 people were awaiting us in the colony's main auditorium when we arrived. The building occupied land that had been part of the cremation ground. Yohei took a seat at the front of the hall, and I sat beside him to take in the atmosphere. With us were the WHO contact in the Maharashtra state government; the president of the colony and a cured leprosy patient, Bhimrao Madhale; Tatsuya Tanami, then the Nippon Foundation executive director responsible for leprosy-control efforts; Kazuko Yamaguchi, the director of the Sasakawa Memorial Health Foundation; and Kanae Hirano, our English-Japanese interpreter.

Seated alongside us was a female graduate school student from the University of Mumbai. The residents and staff members at the colony spoke

Marathi, and the grad student was there to translate between that language and English for Hirano to handle between English and Japanese.

"Good morning," began Yohei when the introductions were complete. Everyone in the audience was listening intently to hear what this visitor from afar had to say. "I have traveled from Japan to be here today. Please raise your hand if you have heard of Japan."

Nearly everyone raised a hand, including the children in attendance.

"That's impressive. Excellent. Next, raise your hand if you know where Japan is."

Only a single hand went up, that of a boy who appeared to be in his early teens.

"Good for you. And where is Japan?"

The boy's answer filtered back through our two interpreters.

"It's a small island east of India."

That was good enough to earn praise from Yohei. We had heard from Madhale that "small children" at the colony attended public schools. That begged the question as to what the older children did. And Yohei was trying to get a feel for the level of education at the colony.

Madhale took us on a tour of the colony after the welcoming ceremony. Men and women of middle age and older sat along a narrow lane that ran between the residents' houses. They were there to greet Yohei. Most of them were missing hands and feet. Yohei greeted each in turn, placing his hands on the stubs of their limbs.

"I can see that you were one handsome man" he'd offer with a smile. Or, "You must have been popular with the guys."

The seemingly innocuous salutations were unfailingly successful in eliciting smiles. The ravage left by leprosy on these individuals included disfigured faces. They cherished memories of their appearance before they contracted the disease. And they welcomed the reminders from this odd visitor.

Madhale took us next to his house, which was larger than the other dwellings. A crowd of children formed in our wake. Yohei stroked their heads and uttered repeatedly the universal Indian greeting, "Namaste."

We admired the numerous copper pans of all sizes that hung on the wall in Madhale's kitchen and that were clearly a source of pride for their owner. Yohei was more interested, however, in seeing whatever toilet facilities were available to the colony residents.

Madhale led us to a public restroom that stood in a broad shoulder above a stinking sewer of a creek. Concrete revetment secured the banks. The restroom had cement-coated walls and presented a surprisingly pristine appearance. It was only accessible, however, by a staircase—surely a struggle for the colony's numerous residents who had walking disabilities.

Yohei inspected each of the four stalls, none of which had a door. The toilets were fairly clean, but the smell was oppressive. I found myself wondering if Madhale hadn't mobilized the residents to clean the toilets for Yohei's visit. The thought hit me that we hadn't seen any litter on our stroll through the colony grounds. I could well imagine that the head of the colony would want to get things shipshape for an important visitor.

"Toilets provide a pretty good glimpse," Yohei commented to me, "of the sanitary stance of a colony," He then turned to Madhale and asked, "How many restrooms do you have here at the colony?"

"Ten. We've got about 200 households, so ten are really not enough. The residents have to wait in line at each of the restrooms in the morning. Everyone is on edge, and fights break out sometimes."

"What do you do with the excrement?"

"We collect it in tanks and release it later into the creek."

"And without any sewage treatment whatsoever," murmured Yohei with a sour face.

"Collecting" was a matter of letting the excrement and urine accumulate in tanks directly beneath the toilets. The colony simply dumped the contents into the creek when the tanks got full.

"Bad sanitation," Madhale acknowledged with a sigh of resignation, "means more disease."

A large group of residents had gathered on the flatness above the creek near the restroom. Standing nearest to us was an elderly woman in a pink shawl. Yohei's eyes locked swiftly on her feet, which, like those of most of the residents present, were bare. Her toes were so disfigured as to be uncountable. Her fingers, meanwhile, had the look of wire that had been bent with pliers at bizarre angles. Some were missing. Yohei took her hand and struck up a conversation.

"How old are you? And where are you from?"

"I don't remember exactly how old I am. Maybe around 74. I'm here to thank you. I wanted to say 'Thank you' for coming from the far end of Asia to visit our colony."

The woman placed her forehead against Yohei's hand and then pushed the hand back toward him. She looked up at him with an expression that betrayed a curious combination of gratitude and acceptance.

"I got this disease, so my family disowned me, and I came here to live. I've been here for 50 years now. This was forest back then. I cut the trees to sell for lumber and gathered the nuts to sell for food. I worked on the docks loading rice onto ships. I did what I could to survive. But that was then. Look. My hands and feet have become useless. I don't have any interest in living anymore. Still, your visit has filled me with joy."

I took her hands in mine. Her gnarled fingers that remained were lifeless and unresponsive. The skin was as rough as sandpaper. She had conveyed to us something, however, that was inspiring beyond words.

We moved on to another restroom, this one in a square plaza near the center of the colony grounds. It was a study in pungency. Yohei strode right through the buzzing flies to have a look.

The next restroom we found was, like the first, beside the filthy creek. No one had made a show of cleaning any of its six stalls. A statue of a female deity stood in a little Hindu shrine nearby. We heard from Madhale that the sewage-filled creek overflowed frequently in the rainy season, inundating houses. He complained that the state government had been unresponsive to repeated pleas to address this serious problem. This was more for the benefit of the Maharashtra WHO contact, standing beside Madhale, than for us from Japan.

Our Marathi interpreter from the University of Mumbai was struggling mightily to come to terms with what we were witnessing. She broke into tears as she described her feelings.

"I've lived in Mumbai all my life. Yet I had no idea that people in the same city were living in such squalor and misery. I'm ashamed of myself for being unaware."

A twofold problem

An encouraging takeaway from the Sanjay Nagar leprosy colony was something we saw on the other side of the creek. Three cows were grazing there on a spacious expanse of pasture.

"That's a new enterprise for the colony, isn't it?" Yohei asked Madhale.

"Yes, that's right. We started it with funding from a foundation that you established in India. The cows produce milk, which we sell. It's still a small-scale business, but the milk sells well."

Madhale was referring to the Sasakawa India Leprosy Foundation, which Yohei set up in India in 2006. The foundation supports cured leprosy patients in colonies like Sanjay Nagar. It provides small loans to help the cured persons become self-sufficient through business enterprise.

"We plan to grow the herd," reported Madhale with a proud smile.

"You'll become a model colony. Let's take this chance to discuss the issues here, including sanitation, and decide how to proceed with improvements."

Our group headed toward one of the thoroughfares that skirted the colony grounds. We passed numerous individuals along the way who were carrying rolled rush mats under their arms. Yohei stopped and, jutting out his chin, grumbled under his breath.

"They haven't been up front with us here. Those people are just back from begging. Look at those mats. Alms are an easy source of revenue for people at urban colonies like this one. I want the world to be free of beggars. We'll never get rid of discrimination otherwise. People can't raise children properly in poverty."

Yohei patted the heads of the children that were tagging along behind our group. He persisted with his commentary, however, as we continued walking.

"The caste system makes things worse. Parents drag their children into beggary. Children get locked into lives of begging on the street. We end up with a vicious circle of begging and poverty. Breaking that circle is even harder than it looks. Begging is a symbiosis between those in need and those who believe they gain merit by giving alms. Take away the beggars, and you take away the opportunity for gaining merit."

"Here's the temple," interjected Madhale. We had seen the large, rough-hewn wooden figures of the elephant-headed Hindu deity Ganesha and of the revered spiritual figure Sai Baba of Shirdi (died 1918). Immediately to the right of the temple was a meeting hall. Awaiting us there were about 20 men and women, young and old.

Our hosts passed around heavily sugared instant coffee in paper cups. Yohei received a list of 12 issues for the colony and a request for assistance in addressing those issues. The 3 most vexing issues were the needs for securing land rights in the face of urban development, for doing water-control work along the creek to prevent flooding, and for creating jobs for the colony residents.

Madhale and some of the other residents at the gathering revealed a sense of desperation about land rights. The colony had grown impressively over the years. But in the eyes of the law, they were little more than squatters. The owner of the forest land where the colony began had generously permitted their predecessors to live there. But they had never formally secured ownership rights to the real estate. They felt helpless and abandoned and alone. And they were pleading for help.

"This is my second visit to your colony," announced Yohei as he began to address the gathering. "I admire the way you have overcome hardship and accomplished great things here under the leadership of Bhimrao Madhale.

Yohei's voice resonated strongly in the closed hall. He had begun his remarks seated in his chair but stood at this point to continue his remarks.

"India has a lot of colonies that are contending with serious challenges. They have needs similar to those expressed in the requests that I received from you today. Some of your needs are challenges for the state government of Maharashtra to address. Others are challenges that we can help address. For example, installing sewage treatment for the public restrooms here is a job for the state government. So is the task of undertaking flood-control work along the creek.

"As for land rights, we can help. We have gotten the United Nations to take up a resolution that ensures your rights. Did you hear me? The UN General Assembly is about to pass a resolution that calls for recognizing and protecting, in full, your right to lead decent lives."

Yohei raised a document of several pages and told his audience that it was the text of the resolution in question. It carried the title "Resolution on Elimination of Discrimination Against People Affected by Leprosy and Their Family Members." The resolution and an accompanying set of principles and guidelines for fulfilling the resolution had received formal backing from the UN Human Rights Council on September 30. They had subsequently received the approval of the UN General Assembly Third Committee, which handles social, humanitarian, and human rights issues, on November 16. And they would receive unanimous approval in the UN General Assembly on December 21, 2010, five days after our visit to the Sanjay Nagar colony.

"Listen carefully. You have the right to continue living in your colony. Your government will have the responsibility to protect that right. That's all here in this UN resolution. You and we can work together and issue demands based on this resolution to the state government.

"You at this colony are no longer alone in your struggle. You are no longer helpless. We have built an organization of 700 colonies in India called the National Forum. The National Forum makes appeals to state governments on behalf of its member colonies. Formerly, each colony was alone in appealing to its state government. Things are different now. When you need the state government to do something, you have a strong voice to convey your demand. And you have the right. Do you hear me? I'm talking about the difference between making a request and making a demand.

"Leprosy is a twofold problem. The first part of the problem is the medical challenge of curing the disease. The second part is the social challenge of eliminating prejudice and discrimination against persons affected by the disease. We have focused up till now on the medical challenge. But we are on the verge of bringing leprosy under control around the world. And the time has come for putting more effort into tackling the social challenge. We need to shape an environment where patients and cured patients and their family members can enjoy peace of mind.

"Together, let us take our case to the Maharashtra state government. Let us fight for upgrades in the public restrooms, for improvements in education, for the construction of water-control levees, and for the guarantee of property rights. We are already engaged in a similar struggle in the state of Bihar. Our struggle there is for the rights to homes, to land, and to pensions. Bihar has 52 colonies, and the state authorities there are in the final stages of working out measures to resolve the problems. That state is the poorest in India. If we can succeed there, how could we fail here in the far richer state of Maharashtra?

"We encounter the same problems all over the world. You absolutely have the right to the land where you live. You needn't worry. We will work with colonies throughout India to strengthen the National Forum. In our solidarity, we will triumph."

A second miracle

Yohei invited Madhale and the other residents to let him know if they needed any help with documentation for securing property rights. After the gathering dispersed, Yohei sat with Madhale and an elderly resident known as "Chairman" before a portrait of Mahatma Gandhi. Yohei asked about the problem of employment. Chairman replied that lots of residents wanted to work but were unable to find jobs.

"How many people are we talking about?" asked Yohei.

"More than 100," answered Chairman.

"Male or female?"

"Mainly male."

"Have they been to school?"

"Yes, for the most part."

"How many people here go out begging?"

"Maybe 25 or 30 of the 750 residents."

"You've raised an important point. I want to put an end to begging at this colony. That's my goal. So people here have the ability to work but can't get jobs? Is that because they don't get the chance?"

"The leprosy connection is the problem. They apply for jobs, but they get refused because of the leprosy."

Seven or eight residents who had remained in the hall raised hands to show deformed fingers.

"We're over the disease," said one, "but we have these handicaps that prevent us from working."

"Let's agree here today on some concrete measures for addressing problems at hand," proposed Yohei. "Talk with the Sasakawa India Leprosy Foundation about the residents who can't get jobs because of disabilities. The foundation will help with rehabilitation. As for the public restrooms, the director of the Sasakawa Memorial Health Foundation, Kazuko Yamaguchi, is with us here today. And she has promised to resolve the problem. Rest assured that help is on the way."

Yohei then took in hand again the UN resolution that he had waved earlier.

"Do you understand? This is your weapon. Keep this in mind. This UN resolution includes precious guidelines for ensuring your rights as human beings. Those guidelines detail what needs to happen to ensure your dignity and what mustn't happen. Your nation will be a signatory to this resolution. Your government will have pledged to abide by the resolution. To be sure, a UN resolution is not legally binding. Laws don't provide penalties for failing to abide by a resolution. But your government officials cannot look the other way when you pull out this document.

"Do you see what I am saying? You need to remember that this resolution is your weapon. I have copies of the original for those of you who can read English. But get the document translated into Marathi. Have the resolution ready at all times, and use it as necessary to combat discrimination. Foster a strong awareness of the resolution in your community. Keep a copy in each of your homes in the kitchen or on a wall somewhere so that you'll see it every day. Recite it aloud for the members of the community who cannot read.

"Remember that I am with you in your struggle. Your fight is my fight as long as I live. I will never give up the struggle. Let us carry on the fight together."

This stirring call to action in the spirit of common cause elicited vigorous applause. Members of the audience whose legs were barely functional somehow pulled themselves up to acknowledge Yohei's remarks.

I realized anew that, in my travels with Yohei, I was witnessing a historic watershed. The struggle to which Yohei had dedicated his life was unprecedented. That struggle was on the verge of bringing leprosy under control worldwide. But it was more than a medical quest. The struggle was also a fight against the discrimination occasioned by leprosy. That discrimination dates at least since the time of the Old Testament. Ironically, the disparaging biblical references to "lepers" probably don't even refer to the disease that we know as leprosy. No skeletons from the biblical milieu—neither Old Testament nor New—have revealed any evidence of the disease. The biblical anecdotes presumably concern disorders other than leprosy as presently defined. They nonetheless established the dreadful pattern for unfounded discrimination that persisted across millennia.

The struggle against leprosy has, in the past century, yielded a genuine miracle more compelling than any biblical parable. We read tales in the Bible of Jesus curing a single person who had contracted leprosy and a group of such persons. Those tales lose their luster, however, amid the implications of historical findings. Jesus probably never encountered, much less cured, anyone affected by the disease that we know as leprosy. The real therapeutic miracle in vanquishing leprosy began in the mid-20th century with the deployment of the sulfone drugs promin and dapsone and continued with the deployment in the 1980s of multidrug therapy.

Now, Yohei was eyeing a second miracle. He was taking part in a global campaign to eliminate discrimination against persons presently or formerly afflicted by the disease and against their family members. Leprosy-related discrimination was something that neither the Buddha nor Jesus nor any other great religious figure had tackled. But here was Yohei, a visitor from halfway around the world, emboldening the colony residents to demand their rights. He flourished evidence for all to see that the United Nations had guaranteed those rights. And he urged the residents to carry the fight for their rights to their state government and to their national government.

Cured leprosy patients in Bihar had won recognition for their residential land rights. Yohei had brought them to meet the state health minister and other state officials, and the cured persons had taken the opportunity to press their claims directly. The National Forum, launched at Yohei's initiative in 2005, was fortifying the colonies' influence through networking. And the Sasakawa India Leprosy Foundation was providing support to improve living standards in leprosy communities.

A funeral for a slum youth

We hurried from the Sanja Nagar leprosy colony to our next stop, a hospital in Mumbai's Dharavi slum. Dharavi is the second-largest slum in Asia, after Karachi's Orangi. Yohei wanted to pay his respects to a young man he had heard about at the colony. The young man was an activist who had contracted leprosy, had overcome the disease, and had gone on to fight for the rights of others affected by leprosy. Alas, he lost his fight with ailments that arose from aftereffects of his leprosy and died shortly before we arrived.

Yohei met and talked with the physician who had tended to the young man, a woman of 40 something. She led us up to the roof of the hospital for a view of Dharavi. Seen from above, the slum was a sea of roofs of rusting corrugated metal bifurcated by a multilane road. The physician pointed toward a section of the sea and spoke.

"His family's house is down there somewhere."

"And now he's gone," Yohei murmured while turning his eyes toward the former neighborhood of the departed.

"Yes. He fought hard for the rights of those affected by leprosy. It's a shame."

"How many people live in Dharavi?"

"Something like 650,000. I don't know for sure. We hear that the population density is 31,400 people per square kilometer."

"Amazing."

"The population includes some 100 ethnic groups. But most of the residents are Dalits."

"How many leprosy patients do you have here at this hospital?"

"We have about 40 who are presently receiving treatment, including cured patients who are receiving treatment for aftereffects. The young man we lost today had been one of their number."

"He was still young."

"Yes. I hate to lose any patient but especially one so young."

"Will he get a funeral?"

"It ought to be getting under way right now. Would you like to go?"

Yohei, of course, wanted to go. The physician led us down a broad avenue lined with uninviting residences. The buildings, though vertical, were less multistory than single-story hovels piled one atop another. Some looked as if they could collapse at any moment.

Most of the households ran shops. A lot of them had arrayed stacks of large- and small-mouthed earthenware pots fired reddish brown at low temperatures. Some were selling leather goods, some embroidered goods. We came upon a narrow alley between the buildings that obliged us to stoop to pass.

"Here it is," the physician alerted us just after we had entered the alley.

On our left was a small, windowless shanty. We could make out in the dark interior the figures of a grieving couple that we took for the young man's parents. The building, like most of the Dharavi residences that we had passed, was no more than about 10 square meters. It was home, apparently, to 8 or

10 people. Yohei crouched to enter the room but he stopped suddenly at the sound of crying from somewhere up the alley. He told me to go ahead to the funeral and that he'd join me after paying his respects to the parents. When I hesitated, he pushed my back and urged me on.

A few steps took me to an open, brick-paved space that ordinarily served, I could see, as a communal workshop. On the perimeter of the space were piles of the familiar reddish-brown pots. I spotted a well. The crying was that of women. They had formed a line and were entering and exiting a small brick room one at a time. The women turned and cast indifferent looks at me through swollen eyes. Not knowing what to do, I placed my hands together and bowed.

I saw that smoke was rising from a chimney atop the brick room and realized that this was where they cremated their dead. That came as a surprise. Wealthy Hindus, I knew, would spend large sums to have deceased family members cremated in the city of Varanasi (Benares) and the ashes entrusted to the Ganges. My understanding, however, was that those too poor to afford firewood commonly dispensed with cremation and simply disposed of the corpses in the river. The sound of Yohei's voice from behind jostled me out of my rumination.

"Ah, so this is where they do the cremating. Do they do it in that building."

"Looks like it."

"Go have a look."

"Me? I'm not sure I should."

I stood motionless. For this visitor of another nationality and another faith to peer in at a corpse out of curiosity struck me as disrespectful. Yohei, giving up on me, walked over to the brick room briskly, grasped both hands of each woman, surveyed the interior of the room carefully, and returned to the spot where I remained. Looking at me with his characteristically big-eyed gaze, he said nothing about what he had seen inside the brick room and talked instead of what he had heard from the parents.

"I asked how they made their living. They told me that they have another son and that he makes money for the family by selling water at the train station. They said that he makes about 3,000 rupees a month—about ¥5,500 (around $65)—and that they don't receive a single rupee of assistance from the state government."

Yohei's voice betrayed a combination of indignation and sadness. He was recoiling at the social abandonment born of the caste system. As we returned to the avenue by which we had come, I looked into the young man's house. I saw the dirt floor and the cramped space; the bed covered with a simple colored sheet; the mother and grandmother sitting on the bed; the father sitting on the floor, his arms around his knees. They had exhausted their tears and merely hung their heads in silence. I could see that the grandmother had also suffered from leprosy. She had presumably been cured of the disease, but she had lost all her toes, and her feet were swollen and disfigured. I barely managed to suppress the vocal outburst of dismay that welled up inside my throat. The resistance that I had felt at looking in on the cremation under way in the brick room had faded. None of the survivors in the young man's house had the energy to care or even notice our presence. I recalled how the women in line at the cremation had been indifferent to our approach. They, too, had been too grief-stricken to respond one way or another to our presence.

We could see from the outpouring of grief that the young man, a person cured of leprosy, had earned a wealth of love and affection. The downtrodden members of the Dalit castes, I realized, were loyal to one another to the end. Members of other castes who contracted leprosy would likely suffer estrangement from their families. They certainly wouldn't receive funerals when the time came.

Self-help enterprise. And begging.

We grabbed a late lunch after the funeral and headed for the second leprosy colony on our Mumbai itinerary. An hour's drive through the city's insane traffic took us to the Panvel colony, east of Mumbai. Yohei was visiting Panvel for the first time. The colony consists of two rows of small, barrack-like buildings on either side of a tangle of rail lines. Corrugated metal sheathed the buildings. A scraggly stand of trees, possibly oaks, offered something in the way of shade. The bare land around the rail lines was more spacious than seemed necessary. Heat waves rose from the rusting metal tracks in the escalating sunlight.

The Panvel colony was home, we learned, to 150 residents in 28 households. Daily life there meant crisscrossing the railway tracks and the lunar landscape to get from building to building. I shuddered at the thought of the psychological ramifications for the residents. In comparison, the Sanjay Nagar colony had been a paradise. Panvel was reassuring, however, in one respect. It occupied state land, and the residents enjoyed peace of mind in regard to their rights to continue living there in perpetuity.

Our hosts applied red bindi dots to our foreheads and led us to the workshop. The workshop was small but neat and clean. It is a production enterprise supported by a Christian organization. Cured leprosy patients who have disabling aftereffects of the disease earn their livings there making household disinfectant and apparel. They work in several teams. Shyra, the leader of a team that produced disinfectant, talked with Yohei about the work.

"Our team has 13 women."

"How many bottles of disinfectant do you produce each month?" Yohei asked while observing the activity in the workshop.

"We produce 500 a month. And we get 30 rupees a bottle."

"So your disinfectant alone brings in 15,000 rupees a month, right?"

"That's right."

The residents were securing regular income through their hard work, but they remained well below the poverty line.

"Are you a cured patient?" Yohei asked Shyra.

"No. Neither my husband nor I have ever contracted leprosy, but this woman has. This is my mother-in-law."

Shyra gestured toward an elderly woman sitting beside her in a chair. The woman's hands and feet were disfigured.

"She lived in a village about five kilometers from here. The villagers drove her out when she came down with the disease."

Yohei crouched down and, grasping the woman's hands, asked her a question.

"How long ago did you come here?"

"About 40 years ago."

"All the elderly residents here came after being driven out of their villages," added Shyra. "No one in the vicinity knew about this colony for a long time."

"So this was a secret sanctuary," nodded Yohei.

Elderly persons accounted for a conspicuously large percentage of the residents. Among them, we saw missing hands and feet, a nose nearly gone, eyeballs that had disintegrated. Conversely, children accounted for several members of Shyra's workshop team. Their smiling faces and their wonderment at the first-time encounter with Japanese were irresistibly endearing. They reminded me anew of the miracles that the development of a cure for leprosy had wrought.

"Friends," began Yohei in addressing everyone in the workshop, "you have taken your destinies into your own hands. That is amazing. I have visited lots of leprosy-care facilities in this nation, but I have never before seen such impressive effort in the spirit of self-reliance as I have seen here today. I will work with Shyra to secure more assistance for the elderly residents here. In the meantime, here is $500, a token of my admiration for your self-help efforts. Please carry on in your admirable spirit of self-reliance."

Yohei then turned to the children and asked them what they wanted to be when they grew up. Hands shot up, and the young ones voiced their dreams excitedly in turn.

"I want to be a schoolteacher!" "I want to be a cricketer!"

The answers continued in that vein until a boy of around 10 volunteered a response that took Yohei's breath away.

"I want to grow up soon and help my parents."

Yohei, visibly moved, regained his composure and praised the boy for his parental piety. He then called on everyone in the workshop to gather for a group photo. Yohei took the opportunity, however, to gain some crucial insight into how the leprosy colony was actually working.

"Do you know someone who lives here who you'd like to have in the photo but who can't get around on their own? For example, do you know someone who can't participate in things because they can't walk?"

"Yes, yes!" the kids responded immediately. "We have a man here who can't get out of his room."

"Could you take me to see that man?"

"Sure. Let's go!"

The youths took Yohei by the hand and set off with him at a trot. Yohei knew that the Maharashtra state officials with us were eager to display their good work. Foundations under Yohei's oversight were the main sources of funding for the leprosy-control work in the state, and the officials naturally wanted him to see that they were using the funding effectively. That meant inviting Yohei's attention to the self-help teams that plied the workshop. And it meant diverting his attention from the sort of resident that the children were about to introduce.

"Here," announced Yohei's guides. "He's here."

They had delivered Yohei to one of a group of hovels assembled from scraps of wood and corrugated metal. The hovels stood in the woods, somewhat apart from the main buildings of the compound. Yohei needed to crouch to get a look under the low roof, and I did likewise to peer in from behind. Inside, a man was reclining on a board covered with no more than a thin sheet.

"This guy has come from Japan," shouted the children. "Come out and say 'Hello.'"

The man squirmed as if to get his torso upright. Yohei saw, however, that he was missing hands and feet and sought to put him at ease.

"Just as you are!"

Yohei crawled into the hovel, and I crawled in behind. The man had managed to attain a seated posture. His eye sockets were little more than bare bone, his eyes clearly nonfunctional. Yohei stroked the man's legs, which ended at the ankles, and looked up at the man inquisitively.

"Do you have prostheses? Do you have anything to put here?"

"Over there," said the man in a low voice as he nodded toward a corner.

The sunlight that filtered in through gaps in the walls revealed a pair of artificial feet. The prostheses, standing neatly, were more lifelike in the sunlight than the man's own limbs. I wondered if they were a benefit of largesse by Yohei's Sasakawa Memorial Health Foundation. That organization provides financial assistance for the production of prostheses for leprosy patients and cured patients, as well as for orthopedic surgery and for other medical needs. Some leprosy colonies, incidentally, have on-site workshops that produce prostheses.

Yohei sat down beside the man on the makeshift bed and placed an arm around the man's shoulders.

"Your eyes. . . . What's happened to your eyes? Can you see?"

"I can't see."

"Did you take medicine? You've gotten rid of the disease, haven't you?"

"I've been cured of the disease, but my body. . . ." The man nodded down at what was left of his anatomy. "My body won't recover."

"Do you live alone?"

"All alone. But the people here are kind and take care of me. That's how I survive."

"When did you come down with the disease?"

"The symptoms started appearing 15 years ago. Until then, I was living with my family in my hometown, about 300 kilometers from here."

"Did the villagers evict you?"

Yohei had learned that speaking in unvarnished tones is the best way to communicate with people in desperate straits. The man, however, went silent. Yohei closed his eyes and lowered his head and maintained that posture wordlessly for an extended spell.

We heard the voice of an elderly woman outside. We crawled out of the hovel, and Yohei, finding the woman seated on a tree root, took a seat beside her. Her hands and feet were nominally intact, but her fingers were splayed haphazardly, and she was missing all the toes but the big one on her right foot. The children listened respectfully to the exchange, seated on the ground in a ring around Yohei and the woman. I recalled the expression of parental piety by one of their number. And I wondered how their experience at the colony would shape their future attitudes and action in dealing with elderly disabled persons.

"This corner of the grounds was originally a cemetery," the woman informed Yohei.

"Are you still working?"

Yohei had taken the woman's hands in his as they spoke. She clearly appreciated the interest that he displayed, but her countenance darkened as she answered.

"We have a temple near here. I go there twice a week to receive alms."

"How much do you get each day there?"

"I guess somewhere between 10 and 15 rupees. People sometimes give me food."

"So they do have begging here," Yohei muttered to me with a touch of dejection. "Even here at a colony that's a model of self-help enterprise. And this old woman is surely not the only one."

We could but wonder if some of the children seated around us didn't also go out and beg for alms. Yohei and the rest of us carried that doubt with us as we rose, thanked our hosts, and departed the Panvel leprosy colony.

A hero of the movement

Our vehicles, furnished by WHO, carried us next to the city of Pune, about 170 kilometers south of Mumbai. We climbed the mountain highway up the Deccan Plateau at breakneck speed and arrived at our hotel at 6:20 p.m. Pune lies at an elevation of about 600 meters on the western edge of the plateau. It is the second-largest city in the state of Maharashtra, after Mumbai, and is a center of manufacturing and scientific research. We had traveled there for Yohei to attend an international leprosy workshop and to visit a leprosy colony in the city.

Pune provided a lovely setting for the workshop. Our hotel occupied a verdant setting, and we woke to a cool breeze and the sound of birds singing. The workshop kicked off that morning in our hotel's conference hall under the banner "An Inclusive Society: Leprosy and Human Rights." Among the attendees were representatives of nations where leprosy remains a serious problem. We heard reports from them about progress in fighting the disease in Bangladesh, Brazil, Colombia, Ethiopia, Indonesia, the Republic of Korea, and the Philippines, as well as in our host nation of India. Each of the delegates greeted Yohei warmly, shaking hands and exchanging hugs.

Representing Brazil was Cristiano Torres, who had been cured of leprosy. Brazil was then the only nation that hadn't attained the WHO's elimination benchmark of 1 leprosy case per 10,000 population.

"We don't want sympathy," declared Torres on behalf of everyone affected by leprosy. "We want a chance."

On hand from Indonesia was Adi Yosep, a 31-year-old who had been cured of leprosy. Adi appeared as the representative of a nonprofit organization that supports networking among persons who have been cured of leprosy. A youthful Indian who had been cured of leprosy admitted to engaging in begging. He offered a convincing reason, however, for engaging in the practice.

"Lots of Indians afflicted by leprosy beg for alms. So I do, too. It's an opportunity to share information and promote networking among the beggars."

We renewed acquaintances at the workshop with Dr. P. K. Gopal, a hero in the global fight against leprosy. Gopal is a person who has been cured of leprosy and is a cofounder of the International Association for Integration, Dignity and Economic Advancement (IDEA), an advocacy group for persons affected by leprosy. He was instrumental, too, in building the National Forum and led that organization as its chairman until 2014. Yohei and Gopal were soulmates of long standing in the antileprosy crusade, and Yohei had turned to Gopal to take charge of bringing to fruition his initiative for what became the National Forum. I knew Gopal, meanwhile, on account of having interviewed him in Tokyo.

The remarkable Gopal was born into a weaving household in 1941 in the Erode district of the southern Indian state of Tamil Nadu. He was the eldest son among seven children. Symptoms of his leprosy first appeared when he was 12, but he didn't receive prompt treatment. Gopal finally received a formal diagnosis while he was studying economics at a university in Erode. That led to hospitalization and treatment and to recovery. His only aftereffects from the disease are slight disfigurement in the fingers on both hands and numbness in the soles of his feet.

Gopal went to work after graduation as a case worker at Sacred Heart Hospital, a leprosy-care facility in the Tamil Nadu city of Kumbakonam and spent 25 years there. That straddled a 2-year leave of absence to earn a master's degree in medical social work from Loyola College, in Chennai. Sacred Heart opened India's first rehabilitation center for persons who had been cured of leprosy while Gopal was at Loyola, and he became the head of the center on returning to the hospital.

At the rehabilitation center, Gopal worked systematically in tackling challenges inherent to the social framework for persons affected by leprosy: rebuilding the relationships between cured persons and their families, reshaping attitudes in the villages that had expelled persons who had contracted leprosy to accommodate their return after being cured, providing support for education and economic self-reliance. He earned a doctorate in social science from Ranchi University in 1993, and his doctoral thesis centered on the logical framework he had developed for the social rehabilitation of persons cured of leprosy.

The professional and social stature that Gopal attained is extremely rare, of course, for a cured leprosy patient. It is a tribute to the love and devotion that his parents displayed in standing by their son through his struggle. Gopal, incidentally, long refrained from mentioning his medical history to colleagues and other acquaintances. The occasion for his "coming out" was the 14th International Leprosy Congress, held in 1993 in Orlando, Florida. A forum at that gathering featured presentations by persons who had been cured of leprosy and who were revealing their medical histories publicly for the first time, and Gopal participated in the forum as an Indian representative. That led to his participating in launching IDEA the next year in Brazil and to his spearheading the subsequent launching of IDEA India and becoming its first president.

Coming out instilled in Gopal a redoubled passion for his mission. He visited leprosy colonies throughout India while continuing to supervise the care of persons who had been cured of leprosy at the rehabilitation center. Gopal lobbied government agencies, medical organizations, and nonprofit organizations assiduously. He mobilized them to help shape a social environment that would remind persons who had been cured of leprosy of their human dignity and that would prompt them to assert their human rights. Gopal also convened gatherings of persons cured of leprosy to propagate networking and mutual encouragement. He described for us the changes that his work had brought about.

"Leprosy patients and cured patients in India formerly didn't recognize the discrimination against them as a violation of their human rights. They tended to accept it as their fate. Now, they stand up for their rights. Meanwhile, nearly all of the states in India had laws on the books that discriminated against persons affected by leprosy. Most of those states have repealed those laws."

Gopal had thus achieved huge successes. But deeply ingrained attitudes die hard. Witness the difficulty he experienced in holding a forum for cured patients in the impoverished state of Odisha in southeast India. That was in June 2003.

The residents of a leprosy colony and Gopal had brought their proposal for a forum to a local nonprofit organization, and the representatives of the organization had proposed a dilapidated, abandoned building as the venue.

The overtly discriminatory stance evinced by the nonprofit was too much for the colony residents and Gopal to bear, and they negotiated for a more satisfactory venue. Their persistence initially won a tentative concession: the nonprofit would arrange for them to use an aging public hall for the forum. The hall's administrators rejected that plan, however, huffing indignantly that they weren't about to host "a gathering of beggars." At the end of the day, Gopal had no choice but to abandon his plans for a forum in Odisha.

"I'm always thinking of Mahatma Gandhi," Gopal told me in our Tokyo interview. "He'd be at a crucial juncture in negotiating India's independence with his British counterparts, and he'd stand up suddenly in the middle of the negotiations and walk out of the room. He knew that the downtrodden people of India, including those affected by leprosy, were waiting eagerly for his comments [on the progress of the talks]. The downtrodden were always first and foremost in his mind. And he always made time for them, no matter what the circumstances were. His example has been an inspiration to me in my work."

Gopal had left the Sacred Heart rehabilitation center to nurture solidarity in India's leprosy-affected community through Yohei's National Forum initiative. Yohei knew that Gopal was the perfect person for the job. He had instructed Gopal to begin by conducting a survey to get a grasp of all the leprosaria in India, and he had pledged to provide whatever funding was necessary to carry out the survey.

The survey work that Gopal initiated in 2005 soon identified more than 700 leprosaria throughout India. Yohei fulfilled his promise, providing funding through the Nippon Foundation and the Sasakawa Memorial Health Foundation. The National Forum held a growing range of forums nationwide to propagate dialogue between the leprosaria and local nonprofit organizations. Its networking transformed the leprosaria into a powerful, unified force for lobbying the state and national governments. The National Forum had been especially effective in securing pensions for persons who had been cured of leprosy.

Gopal has become the Indian face of the movement for eradicating discrimination against persons affected by leprosy and restoring their rights. India's government recognized his contributions to that movement in 2012 with the nation's fourth-highest civilian award, the Padma Shri.

At the Pune workshop, Gopal and the other participants discussed such issues as how to leverage their strengths through cooperation and how to support the antileprosy movement in the most needy nations. Everyone was excited, of course, about the promising implications of the impending adoption by the UN General Assembly of the leprosy resolution. Yohei, in his remarks to the gathering, launched a familiar appeal.

"Leprosy is a twofold problem," he began in a replay of his comments at the Sanjay Nagar colony. "The first part of the problem is the medical challenge of curing the disease. The second part is the social challenge of eliminating prejudice and discrimination against persons affected by the disease. We have made a lot of progress in tackling the medical challenge. Now, the official backing from the United Nations will stimulate progress in tackling the second part of the problem, the prejudice and discrimination.

"Researchers and health care professionals have led the work in addressing the medical side of the problem. Leprosy patients and cured patients need to take the lead in addressing the issue of prejudice and discrimination. They need to reach out to one another and join hands across national and regional borders in a united effort. They need to pool their experience and knowledge and thereby maximize their collective influence.

"I was at a leprosy colony yesterday in Mumbai where the residents described feeling helpless and alone. But I assured them that they are not helpless, that they are not alone. I could offer that assurance because of the UN resolution and because of the solidarity that is taking shape in our movement at the national level and at the global level.

"Each person in our movement needs to understand the principles and guidelines that accompany the UN resolution and cite them effectively in negotiating with government agencies. That will help bring about positive change. Each individual needs to come to terms with their rights and with their human dignity. Each individual needs to take the initiative in asserting those rights and that dignity."

Yohei emphasized to the gathering the importance that he attached to putting an end to begging through enterprise and self-reliance. He noted that the Sasakawa India Leprosy Foundation, established in 2006, was funding 72 self-help projects at leprosy colonies across India. And he called on the Indian participants to take part in broadening the range of such projects. He also called for maintaining pressure on the government to secure pensions and suitable living accommodations for severely disabled and cured elderly persons who cannot work.

In the afternoon, we visited the Anandwan leprosy colony, in the Dapodi district of northern Pune. Anandvan dates from 1952 and is one of India's larger leprosy colonies, accommodating some 400 people in 110 households. It was like the Panvel colony, which we had visited the previous day, in that it straddled rail lines. The land under the colony belonged to a railway public corporation, and that ownership had apparently engendered a sense of security about residential rights. Among the facilities at the colony were a modest library, a medical clinic, and—a sight that warmed Yohei's heart—a flour mill. The mill verified that self-help enterprise was taking hold. Our hosts reported that plans were under way for dairy farming at the colony.

Enlivening the scene were the colorful saris worn by female residents. Male residents assembled around the women in a perhaps chivalrous move at barricading. The effort was futile, however, in the open space where the residents had gathered by way of welcome. Birds flitted about, as if to flout any notions of exclusion.

A donation of $1,000 from Yohei drew applause. The leader of the colony signed a receipt for the largesse and pledged to discuss with the residents how to use the funds. His fingers on both hands were shrunken, and he grasped the pen between a stiff thumb and a misshapen index finger. Signing the receipt thus took a fair bit of time, but Yohei waited patiently and smilingly insisted on a handshake when the signing was done.

2

AFTER THE SANDSTORM
CAIRO AND ALEXANDRIA

Yohei could sleep anywhere. For him, airport layovers were opportunities for napping and, having secured sufficient slumber, reading. That's how I'd assumed he'd spend our four-hour wait at Dubai International Airport. We had landed there at midnight after taking a 10:25 p.m. flight from Mumbai on 12 December 2010.

As far as the eye could see were tax-free shops vending luxury goods. I chose to loosen my petrified bones by walking briskly up and down the broad mezzanine corridors that stretched overhead. On returning after several round trips, I expected to find Yohei seated with a book, his legs anchoring a suitcase. He was nowhere, however, to be seen. As I began to search for my companion, a voice called my name from behind.

"Hey, why don't you join me here?"

Seated on the carpet, Yohei riveted me with flashing eyes that recalled his father's famous gaze. When I declined the invitation, he rolled over, resting his head cheek in hand. I began to regret not having secured a room for him to get some proper rest.

"We saw a lot of beggars in Mumbai, didn't we?" Yohei mulled. "I want to know what they're thinking, why they can't do something else."

Even in the middle of the night, the 24-hour airport pulsed with the comings and goings of Westerners and Arabs. Yohei looked up at them intermittently. I was getting sleepy and sat down in a chair comfortably removed from him and closed my eyes.

The boarding time neared. Yohei came over to where I was sitting. He was visibly excited about something.

"I've got it!" he blurted out with a childlike glee at discovery. "I've figured out how the beggars feel. Sitting there on the floor, I was at a completely different eye level from that of the people passing by. So I wasn't the least bit self-conscious. All I saw was the people's feet. And the people passing by took no notice of me. I can perfectly well imagine taking the next step and asking for alms. They say that if you do it for three days, you'll never quit. And I understand that perfectly, now. You're not the least self-conscious, and if you can get some cash that way, then why not?"

Yohei was 71 years old. He had on the same Indian outfit of white cotton that he'd been wearing since we were in Mumbai.

"If I'd've had an empty can in front of me," he laughed, "someone surely would have dropped in some change."

Yohei flew business class, and we had the run of airports' VIP lounges. That was to be expected for the WHO goodwill ambassador for the elimination of leprosy and Japan's ambassador for the human rights of people affected by leprosy. Yohei didn't really care how he traveled, however, as long as he reached his destinations for fulfilling his mission.

Our plane departed after a delay of nearly two hours. We landed at Cairo International Airport at 8 a.m. We grabbed breakfast at the hotel we'd booked and then boarded a bus, lunch boxes in hand, without pausing to rest in our rooms. We were headed for a sanatorium somewhere "across the desert." Behind us was another bus. Joining us on the journey were journalists from local media. The Egyptian people knew essentially nothing about leprosy. Yohei, through the WHO, had mobilized the media in the name of raising awareness of the reality of the disease.

Cairo's traffic was even worse than the horror stories we'd heard. On working our way clear of the city at long last, we were in the desert, headed northwest. Also cutting across the desert was a railroad line. Our bus stopped before crossing the tracks, though not so much as a signal marked the crossing.

In the distance, an incongruous form appeared, bug like, between the cloudless sky and the skin-colored desert landscape. I wondered if some Egyptian statute obliged drivers to stop for a train, no matter how distant it might be, and to wait for it to pass before proceeding, however long a wait that might entail. Our driver, seemingly accustomed to the train waits, folded his arms across the steering wheel and, after a while, buried his face in his arms.

The freight train teased us with its lugubrious approach. Astounded at the prodigious length, I began to count the cars, but I abandoned the exercise as the number swelled. This was not a matter of a mere 10 or 20 carriages. I felt as if some sort of a massive structure, like a seawall, was edging across the sand.

The ties lay submerged in the sand, the rails barely visible above, pulsing up and down under the onslaught of steel wheels.

"Cairo's a big and crowded place," noted our guide, a handsome WHO physician by the name of Abraham. "Compared with Cairo's urban congestion, the sanatorium where we're headed is quiet and peaceful, a decent place to live. The current head took over three years ago and has turned the sanatorium into an excellent facility."

Abraham provided a basic summary of the sanatorium. Built in 1932, it started out as a public-sector hospital for the forced, lifelong isolation of people who had contracted leprosy. It presently houses about 700 patients who have leprosy or who have recovered from the disease but are contending with its aftereffects or with related secondary ailments. The breakdown by gender is 65% male and 35% female, and the hospital has separate quarters for the males and females.

Yohei, wearing sunglasses, listened quietly to the explanation. This was his first visit to a leprosy sanatorium in Egypt. Securing visitation access to leprosariums is difficult in the Islamic world, with the notable exception of Indonesia.

Egypt had brought leprosy largely under control by 1994. At the end of 2009, registered sufferers in the nation numbered just 912, and the prevalence of leprosy was 0.13 per 10,000 population. The disease has proved more intractable in Egypt's upper-Nile region than in the delta population centers of Cairo and Alexandria. Leprosy reportedly remains a problem in five upstream districts.

An expanse of greenery appeared suddenly on the far side of the desert and broadened with our approach. We were soon in the midst of a grove of cacti. Looking up at the fat, towering plants, I neglected to ask what in the world anyone was doing with so many cacti there, but Abraham panegyrized them in the clear timbre of a minstrel. "Who'd believe," he mused rhetorically, "that apples would grow on cacti?" I didn't know what to make of his musing, whether he was citing a passage from literature or whether he was simply joking spontaneously. For lack of a better response, I simply offered a forced smile.

Nearly three hours had passed since we left Cairo. The cacti completely covered the land along both sides of the road. Visible nearby, meanwhile, was a mango orchard. On emerging from the greenery, we came upon the palace-like architecture of the Abu Zaabal leprosarium. The buildings evoked an imposing majesty that belied their age.

The sorrow of no return

December was consistent with the year-round pattern of rainless weather in Egypt's inland climes. The clear sky was cloudless, the air cooler than I had expected. Occasional gusts of wind carried payloads of sand. A boy, clinging to a crutch, sat on a bench in the spacious garden in front of the main gate. He appeared to be in his midteens and had lost a leg. This, surely, was not our welcoming party. Yohei hurried over to the bench as soon as he disembarked from the bus and sat down beside the boy.

"Show me your leg," Yohei urged deferentially. He reached out and touched the limb that the boy raised and peered into the youth's unsmiling face. "You'll be all right," Yohei assured the boy. "This leg won't get any worse. Do you have a prosthetic leg? You're over the disease, right?" The boy, possibly intimidated by the reporters and their video cameras and still cameras, said nothing. Yohei turned to the journalists and, clearly conscious of the broader audience that they served, issued a veritable proclamation.

"This boy contracted leprosy, but effective drug treatment has cured his disease completely. Look, I can sit here beside him and touch him, and I am in no danger of contracting the disease. Please understand. Leprosy is not genetic. Nor is it very contagious. Do any of you still believe that leprosy is divine punishment? It is not. Leprosy is an infectious disease caused by the namesake bacillus. It is a curable disease. It is anything but divine punishment."

Sanatorium patients sat chatting under the rich verdure of large trees on benches scattered across the entryway garden. The complex beyond included a tall building that I guessed to be the sanatorium headquarters and residential-style buildings that housed examination and treatment facilities, inpatient wards, and dormitories. Amid the singing of birds in the arboreal greenery, the setting was every bit as peaceful as Abraham had promised.

Embellishing the acoustic backdrop was a peculiar sound that was more turkey gobble than songbird aria. Each spurt of gobbling started forcefully and tailed off gradually, ending with an elongated coda. The gobbling voices rose in turn, as if in a musical round. When one exited, another entered.

I soon identified the source of the gobbling in the slightly upraised faces of female residents of the sanatorium. The women had gathered to get a look at Yohei and his entourage. Each had a hijab wrapped around her head and wore garb that provided complete coverage down to her wrists and ankles.

The low-exposure apparel characteristic of rigorously Islamic states conceals the identity of the wearer, but discreetly careful observation revealed most of these women to be well up in years. Extending their lips like a bird's beak, they would then emit a voice while flapping their tongue against both lips. With us was Yoshiaki Sasaki, then a senior research fellow at the Tokyo Foundation, and I queried him about this curious vocalization.

"That's something that women in the Arab world do," Sasaki explained. "They use that vocalization to celebrate weddings, to send off funeral processions, and to welcome special guests, like today. The vocalization expresses a welling over of emotion."

Sasaki had spent time in the department of theology at what was then the University of Libya and was well versed in Islamic culture. "This is a hearty welcome," he avowed, "for Yohei."

The director of the sanatorium appeared before us dressed in clinical white and sporting an amiable smile on a hirsute face. He was visibly taken aback by the large media contingent, but he didn't let that impinge on his dutiful courtesy in greeting the WHO's goodwill ambassador for the elimination of leprosy. And he wasted no time in beginning our tour of his sanatorium facilities.

We learned that the Abu Zaabal leprosarium comprised three areas: a central area occupied by a clinic, pharmacy, and offices and two residential areas for males and females. The clinic, which included a facility for dental care, provided a full regimen of multidrug therapy. Each of the rooms in the residential ward for males had two canopied beds. The furnishings were spare, but the rooms were immaculate.

Some of the residents were unable to walk and observed us at repose. Yohei headed straight for an elderly resident we'd heard had been there for 50 years and, thrusting his face forward, placed his cheek against the man's. Another resident, who we'd heard had been there for 31 years, was missing his left leg below the knee. His right leg, though complete, was conspicuously disfigured.

Yohei asked the second man, who was also elderly, to remove his sock. The man moved to comply, but his hands were mere stumps, devoid of fingers, so Yohei helped. He stroked the leg, which looked as if it had been chewed by some sort of beast, and asked the man about life in the sanatorium.

"I came down with this disease when I was 11 years old," the man replied. "The staff here has taken good care of us all along, so, of course, I am grateful."

Residents who had been cured of the disease but who displayed various aftereffects rested in the tree shade on the promenade outside. One who captured my attention was an elderly man who gave the appearance of having been there for thousands of years. Seated in a wheelchair, he maintained a fixed gaze. I soon realized that he was blind, his eyes a foggy white, unblinking.

Some of the people on the promenade had faces textured with nodules. They reminded me of photos of Saint Damien of Molokai (1840–1889), the Belgian priest who devoted his life to caring for persons afflicted by leprosy in Hawaii and who contracted the disease through his work. I knew that plastic surgery could remove the nodules and wondered if and why the people I saw had resigned themselves to living with the disfigurement.

A resident had seated another in a chair and was giving him a shave. Yohei walked over and asked to be next. When Yohei's turn came, we realized when the barber went to work that he was working without shaving cream. "Ouch!" bellowed Yohei as the barber dragged the razor up across the WHO goodwill ambassador's neck under his chin. "Ouch!!!" Undeterred, the barber next grasped Yohei's head firmly between his hands and, bending it left and then right, shaved both cheeks. The customer emerged from the shave with an impressive portfolio of red scratches as souvenirs of the experience.

In the dormitory next door, we encountered a patient who was receiving the multidrug treatment. Both of his legs had swollen as an adverse reaction to the therapy. Yohei crouched down and rolled up the man's trouser legs. He saw that the calves were swollen tight and immediately began a massage of caressing and rubbing.

"Thank you," effused the man, palpably soothed. "That made me feel a lot better."

"The swelling is a mystery," confided the sanatorium director. He had accompanied us throughout our tour of the facility and was now seated beside Yohei. "The drugs have killed all of his leprosy bacilli."

"Do you have others like this man?"

"Not a lot. But I sense that the multidrug treatment is triggering the emergence of drug-resistant strains of the bacteria."

"You've got to be careful about the balance between the three drugs."

"Yes, you're right. We've got to fine-tune the prescription for each individual."

Two decades had passed since the development of the multidrug treatment for leprosy, and the regimen had earned high regard for its consistent effectiveness in beating back the disease. The sanatorium director was aware, however, of what had occurred with antibiotics in other disease categories. Antibiotics wrought a revolution in fighting bacterial diseases, but the emergence of antibiotic-resistant strains of "superbug" bacteria has diminished the reliability of antibiotics against several diseases.

"Let's head over to the women's area," proposed Yohei.

Outside, the path took us between rows of dwellings and shops suggestive of a small town. Dragonflies danced about in the air, reminding me of the colony we had visited in Pune, India. Residents were relaxing outside under extended awnings, seated in chairs or on the ground.

Yohei stopped in front of an elderly man who was sitting at the entrance to a male residence. The man's right eye was askew and bulging. Yohei sat down and, placing both his hands around one of the man's, struck up a conversation.

"You've lost your sight, haven't you? Where are you from?"

"My home is far away."

"I bet you want to go home."

"No, I don't think of going home anymore. This is the best place for me."

The man peered into the distance with presumably sightless eyes. Yohei maintained his grip on the man's hand, giving no sign of moving on. The journalists had gathered around the two men. A woman from a television station pointed a microphone at Yohei and started asking questions.

"Mr. Sasakawa, why are you so interested in leprosy?"

"Humankind has committed all kinds of errors," Yohei began, turning to the camera without letting go of the man's hand. "The way we have handled leprosy is an especially shameful blot on human history. We've trod on the very humanity of the sufferers of the disease. At the heart of the fight against leprosy is a refusal to accept what isn't right. I've dedicated my life to this fight in that spirit. I want to correct the misperceptions about leprosy and end the prejudice against its sufferers.

"This person's hand is warm," Yohei continued, stroking the man's hand. "Blood courses through his veins. Even holding his hand like this presents no risk of catching the disease. And I want everyone watching on TV to understand something: whatever you have heard or believed about leprosy being divine punishment is absolutely wrong."

"What is the most stubborn obstacle in the fight against leprosy?"

"Discrimination," declared Yohei emphatically, his voice rising. "We haven't made any progress whatsoever in eliminating discrimination."

"Please share a message with us for the Egyptian people."

Yohei complied, turning his face again to the camera.

"First of all, I want you to know that this sanatorium is a wonderful, well-run facility. I also want you to know that leprosy is just another disease, like tuberculosis or cholera. I want you to know, too, that it is not especially contagious and that it is entirely curable when someone contracts the disease. We need to welcome those who have recovered from leprosy back into society. Unfortunately, Egyptians have not done that. So even people who have overcome the disease remain isolated in sanatoriums like this one. That is simply not right."

"But some of the patients say that they don't want to go home even after they have been cured."

"That's the saddest thing of all. They really do want to go home. They want to go home, but they feel that they can't. Why do you think that is so? It's because their families don't welcome them back. I call on all of you to understand the reality of this disease, to abandon your misconceptions, and to welcome these individuals with open arms as fellow members of society, as fellow human beings. I call on you to make the effort to set things right."

A female chorus

We took a bus to the women's area, where we were met by a group of nuns. Some long-term residents were sunning themselves in a well-tended garden.

"This is not so much a hospital," Yohei observed to me after taking in the sight, "as a geriatric home. It's a geriatric home equipped with medical facilities. People who have received attentive care here naturally don't want to go back to the families that threw them out. But that really is unfortunate."

Entering a dormitory room, we saw two empty beds and one on which an elderly woman was reclining. Yohei strolled over to the head of the bed and addressed the woman.

"You look pretty fit."

The woman sat up, hanging her legs over the side of the bed. One of the legs was a prosthesis. Yohei crouched down and began to caress the leg but quickly stopped.

"You don't touch a woman's leg casually," he reminded himself aloud, "in the Islamic world."

The next room we visited also had just a single occupant. We could see in an instant that the woman had suffered severely. Her eyelids were sunken, and we interpreted that as an indication that her eyeballs had deteriorated. All four of her limbs were horribly deformed. She raised her arm, however, to invite a handshake. Yohei took her fingerless hand between his hands and held it firmly against his forehead.

"I love the director here," the woman declared in a songlike voice. "He really, really takes good care of us."

"That's great to hear," replied Yohei. "I want you to live a long life. And when you turn 100, I'll come to celebrate."

"Yay!" Her voice fairly lit up the room.

We stepped out into the garden, where we again heard the gobble-trilling sound of voices. Four or five elderly women, their heads completely concealed in hijabs, were sitting on benches in the tree shade and vocalizing joyfully. A glance at the mouths visible through openings in the hijabs revealed tongues flapping laterally and beating on wide-open lips.

"They call it *zaghareet*," explained Sasaki. "It's something that only women do."

Two women seated on another bench, one cradling a baby and the other holding a somewhat older child, also cut loose with the trilling. Their families had presumably evicted them, along with their children. Yohei walked over and caressed the young ones' skin to check that they had not contracted the disease. Not uttering a word, he then made his way toward another dormitory building.

Yohei made a brief detour, however, over to an elderly woman who was standing beneath a mango tree. That woman, too, launched into the *zaghareet* trilling. She had apparently sensed Yohei's presence without seeing him, for both of her eyeballs had decayed. One of the nuns picked some leaves of basil from the garden and handed them to Yohei. The elderly woman was 70- or 80-something and was wearing Arab garb that concealed her completely. Yohei touched her hand. She pressed her forehead against his hand and spoke through tears. "Your visit has shone a light into our lives. Thank you."

We passed by a grape trellis to reach the next dormitory building. Once again, peculiar voices arose in greeting to Yohei. These were a veritable shrieking and sounded to me like they were enunciating something akin to "Bella, bella, bella." Inside the building were sky-blue walls and two rows of six beds each. Two elderly women were sitting on beds beneath threadbare canopies and chatting. Their expressions brightened at the sight of Yohei. I had been concerned that our party might be seen as dealing with the residents as curiosities. Yet the two women broke into their *zaghareet* welcome even as the TV crew pointed video cameras in their faces in turn and as the still photographers did likewise.

The women were wearing black-rimmed glasses, the lenses of which were as thick as magnifying glasses and distorted the women's eyes beyond recognition. Yohei's expression darkened as he observed the bare feet visible beneath the otherwise all-concealing garments. The feet were so unbelievably swollen that the women seemed to have no ankles. And the skin on the elephantine limbs was rough and devoid of luster.

Back outside, we strolled through the garden. Dominating the scene was a big baobab tree. Women here and there serenaded us with *zaghareet* trilling. A woman was sunning herself beside the tree. She had wrapped her head in fold after fold of black turban, and the sun reflected off her robed torso and legs and projected her face in an exaggerated whiteness. Her eyes, nose, and mouth appeared to lie paper flat on the plane of a ghostlike face. I couldn't be certain whether something had flattened her features or whether the depth of the turban obscured their contours.

All the women seated on the benches launched into a renewed round of trilling and then began singing a song. The Arab world is a realm of singing. Before battle, warriors would improvise poetic lines about vanquishing the enemy and sing them to the tune of a melody also composed on the spot. The women improvised lyrics and a melody for us, too.

> Sasakawa-san is handsome
> Sasakawa-san is handsome
> We are sad at your leaving
> We are sad at your leaving
> Come see us again
> Be sure to come see us again

Yohei turned to address the journalists. That is to say that he turned to address the Egyptian people.

"Leprosy is a curable disease. People of Egypt, please understand that. The sufferers of this disease have historically experienced discrimination. But the United Nations has passed a resolution that calls for eliminating discrimination against people who suffer from leprosy, people who have recovered from the disease, and the families of those people. It calls for recognizing the right of those people to return to society and to work, to study, and to marry, just like all of you. In other words, the resolution calls for recognizing their human rights.

"All the member nations of the United Nations, including Egypt, have ratified the resolution. To be sure, the resolution is not legally binding. It depends on all of you to take effect. So please do your part to translate the ideal expressed in that resolution into reality."

We got back on our bus when we had completed our tour of the leprosarium. Yohei, seated behind me, leaned forward and sighed, "The discrimination is horrible. To think that they would toss out even small children like that…"

A sanatorium like a concentration camp

Historic Alexandria, lauded as the "pearl of the Mediterranean," lies on the seacoast about 200 kilometers north of Cairo. Its lovely cityscape was pretty gritty, the aftereffect of a sandstorm two days before we arrived. The sky was clear, however, and the sunlit sea flashed a cloudy white well into the distance, possibly on account of a high concentration of sand.

We left Cairo at 6:30 a.m. and, heading straight north, reached Alexandria's Amria leprosarium a little before 10:30 a.m. The leprosarium occupies a hilly perch southwest of central Alexandria, where it commands a sweeping vista of the city. Its buildings are former British barracks from the colonial era, partly remodeled for their present purpose, and present the profiles of Quonset huts.

A physician in a white frock escorted us on our tour of the facility. A bit unnerving was a guy in Ray-Ban sunglasses and a leather jacket who kept both hands in his jacket pockets, made no effort to shake hands with us, and maintained a constant distance as he tailed us throughout our tour. The physician identified him as the director of the facility, but the man neither smiled nor made any move to merge with our group.

We heard that the leprosarium had 20 residents. That was down, we learned, from a peak of 200 to 250 about 10 years earlier, but the facility still got about 4 new residents a year. The leprosarium had an on-site clinic and a full-time professional staff of two physicians and six nurses. It was unusual in that all the residents were male; female patients received treatment on an outpatient basis.

The building we visited had no partitions and offered an unobstructed view from front to rear. It had a white tile floor, which gave a hygienic impression but amplified the bracing impact of the cold, dry December air. The five beds were few and far between in the spacious interior. A like number of individuals whose sorry condition belied their alleged status as "cured patients" sprawled on beds or lounged in chairs. Their ethnic garb was that of the nomadic Berber or Bedouin ethnic groups.

An elderly man lay face up, his eyes bulging, his jaw hanging open. Another elderly man had ulcerous patches across both legs that gave the red look of burns. The sores were visible because they had been left unbandaged.

"That's appalling," grumbled Yohei. "You'd think they could at least put some bandages on." Our interpreter, Hirano Kanae, declined to render his complaint into English.

Yet another man had open sores on his legs that were festering. And the scent of pus in the air was surely not attributable solely to any one resident. These patients were simply not receiving treatment for such lesions. The life was gone from their milky-white eyes, and even if the eyes could still see, their owners were blindly unresponsive when Yohei extended a hand.

Yohei found still more cause for concern outside. Men lounged in the shade of trees, their mouths hanging open in the manner of senile dementia.

"This place is like a concentration camp for lifers," Yohei muttered. "Just look at their faces. You don't see a smile anywhere. Those eyes might be able to see, but they're lifeless. You've sort of got to salute the Egyptian government for letting us see such an inhuman facility."

I walked away from Yohei and strolled around the expansive grounds. Residents sat or lay apart from one another under the trees. They were the living dead.

Yohei called me over. He was standing atop a rise at the edge of the grounds and looking out over the city and sea.

"This is a hill of homesickness," Yohei remarked. "Try standing here and gazing out."

He was recalling a tall mound at the Tama Zenshoen leprosarium in a suburban quarter of western Tokyo. Patients there had built the mound. It was the only place in the sanatorium where they could see out over the tall fence of thorny holly.

"Frankly, this has come as a shock," Yohei confessed. "I've done everything possible to put an end to that kind of so-called treatment, and yet..." He kept gazing into the distance as he spoke. "Did you see their eyes? They really are just like people left abandoned in a concentration camp, aren't they? No one is out there to take them back. The staff could at least put some gauze on the open sores.

"We saw a group of three or four people out in the sun, but no one was talking with anyone else. They just stood there silently with blank, blind looks. Those are the eyes of people who have given up hope. They reveal no emotion whatsoever, not even pain or sadness. They no longer even have tears of longing for home. They're just soulless, empty shells."

I listened silently. In the distance, the man in Ray-Bans was staring in our direction. Yohei continued, mincing no words.

"I've been to more than 100 sanatoriums and colonies around the world. And I've never seen anything like this before. It made me shudder. But it was worth the three-hour trip from Cairo. This is not a sanatorium. It's a home for people waiting to die. I'm glad that I got to see that a place like this exists. It's a reminder that I've still got a lot of work to do."

Despair beyond hopelessness

The difference between Egypt and India was all too conspicuous in regard to leprosy. To be sure, expulsion from home and from hometown was long a fate common to sufferers of the disease in both nations. Lots of Indians who had contracted the disease had banded together, however, in building colonies on their own and pursuing communal lifestyles. Egypt's leprosariums, on the other hand, were government-built facilities for isolating individuals who had contracted the disease. And they now served more as geriatric homes than as sanatoriums.

We had visited only two facilities in Egypt, but each exhibited features worthy of note, and those features epitomized opposite ends of the heaven-and-hell spectrum. The unfortunate souls we saw at the Alexandria facility were "inmates," rather than "residents." We were unable to verify the ethnic composition of the patients there, but the apparel suggested that most of them were of nomadic ethnic groups. Whether the patients in Alexandria were receiving any treatment for their disease was unclear. Addressing them elicited only blank looks, inviting the suspicion that the staff might be keeping them sedated.

We surmised that they had been expelled by their communities, that they had then taken up a life of begging in Alexandria, and that the authorities had rounded them up and committed them to the leprosarium. Only one man in the Alexandria facility had responded verbally when addressed by Yohei. Asked if he didn't want to go home, the man replied, "I don't want to go home. I've got no family to go home to." The utterance was so utterly devoid of hope that the voice carried not even a tone of despair. I felt an uncontrollable urge to get away from the place as quickly as possible.

Yohei and I descended the leprosarium's hilly perch and crossed a bridge over a broad swamp formed by water from the sea and a river. Looking back at the leprosarium, I could just make out the semicircular cross-sections of some of the buildings. Yohei, however, averted his gaze from the leprosarium. "Estuary. Brine," he murmured absently. "This has been appalling. Those men don't even gaze out from up there toward the lands roamed by their people. Even if they were to cast a glance homeward, it wouldn't signify any real desire to return home."

We visited the Bibliotheca Alexandrina, which stands on the approximate site of the ancient world's famed Library of Alexandria. Also before leaving Alexandria, we took the opportunity to visit the Suzanne Mubarak Regional Centre for Women's Health and Development (since renamed the Alexandria Regional Center for Women's Health and Development). We then headed for three hours straight back to Cairo.

The next day, we visited Egypt's Ministry of Health and Population and discussed leprosy and issues for medical care in Egypt with an adviser to the minister. We learned that Egypt has 17 treatment centers for leprosy and that several of the centers have traditionally been run by Catholic nuns from overseas.

Yohei and those accompanying him, except me, flew out that night to Beirut. I was unable to join them because I had traveled to Israel a few years earlier, and my passport bore entry and exit stamps from that sojourn. Alas, Lebanon is one of several Arab nations that persist in refusing entry to travelers on passports that carry Israeli stamps.

The stop in Beirut was for Yohei to attend a conference hosted by the WHO's Regional Office for the Eastern Mediterranean. That office, one of six regional WHO platforms, serves North Africa, the Middle East, and West Asia. It covers 22 nations over a west-to-east swath from Morocco to Pakistan. All of those nations have ostensibly brought leprosy under control, but military strife and political instability render suspect the accuracy of the reports from a number of these nations. That includes Lebanon, where civil strife has persisted since the 1970s, and Afghanistan, Iraq, Somalia, Sudan, and Yemen.

3

NOT AS THINGS APPEAR
MALAWI

The Great East Japan Earthquake forced the suspension of overseas trips by Yohei and his colleagues at the Nippon Foundation. It struck on March 11, 2011, three months after our visit to Egypt, and laid waste to a vast swath along Japan's Pacific coast north of Tokyo. The earthquake, the tsunami, and the subsequent disaster at the Fukushima Daiichi Nuclear Power Station occasioned a rethinking of basic assumptions about civilization. Providing all assistance possible to the relief effort commanded the full attention of everyone at the Nippon Foundation.

Yohei's peripatetic work in the fight against leprosy resumed in earnest four months later. We embarked at Narita International Airport on July 12 for Africa. The destinations on our itinerary were Malawi, a small nation in the continent's southeast, and the Central African Republic, which lies just north of the equator.

Our Japan Air Lines flight took us first to Frankfurt Airport, where we had a six-hour-plus layover. We made our way through the labyrinthine route from our gate to the boarding platform for the monorail. Yohei declined, as always, to rely on the mechanical assistance of such contrivances as escalators and moving sidewalks. In Tokyo, he walks up and down the stairs daily to and from his seventh-floor office in the Nippon Foundation Building.

We boarded our flight a few minutes before midnight and arrived at Ethiopia's Addis Ababa Bole International Airport at 7 a.m. From there, we embarked on a flight for Lilongwe International Airport, in Malawi's capital, after a layover of four hours. Yohei was making his second visit to Malawi, having been there 11 years earlier. But I confess that I couldn't even pinpoint the nation on a map when I first heard of our itinerary. Only after some searching did I find it in Africa's lower east, landlocked inland from the coast that faces Madagascar.

39

Malawi, slightly smaller than the state of Pennsylvania, cuts a narrow, vertical profile on the map. Surrounding the nation are Zambia on the northwest, Tanzania on the northeast, and Mozambique on the east, south, and west. Stretching up and down the nation's eastern flank is Lake Malawi, which is the third-largest lake in Africa and ninth largest in the world in surface area. Lake Malawi's 29,600-square-kilometer footprint is nearly as large as Belgium and accounts for more than one-fifth of Malawi's aggregate surface area. The lake abounds in tropical fish and hosts more species of fish than any other lake.

My most powerful initial impression of Malawi was its stunning distance from Japan. The flights had taken 11 hours from Narita to Frankfurt, 7 hours from Frankfurt to Addis Ababa, and 4 hours from Addis Ababa to Lilongwe. Including layovers, the transit time totaled 32 hours. I marveled anew at Yohei's physical and spiritual vitality. We would endure jolting rides on Malawi's rough roads to the leprosy colony where we were bound. Yohei would also hold discussions with the nation's president and minister of health and with WHO officials. And an equally grueling schedule awaited us in the Central African Republic.

I had received vaccinations before leaving Japan for tetanus, diphtheria, hepatitis A, and typhoid fever. The easygoing Yohei had assured me that we didn't need vaccinations for hepatitis B or for malaria, and I had reluctantly accepted his assurance. Hepatitis B, he had insisted, was not a big concern. Yohei had acknowledged that malaria was a real risk but had noted that we would be traveling with people from the WHO and that they would be able to provide us with medicine in the event of infection.

Malawi is in the southern hemisphere, so our July arrival was in midwinter. That and the elevation, higher than 1,000 meters, rendered tropical diseases unlikely. The equatorial clime of the Central African Republic, however, meant that country would be swarming with disease-bearing mosquitoes.

Addis Ababa Bole International Airport occupies an elevation of 2,334 meters. A light rain was falling when we boarded our plane, and our breath was white in the chilly air. The rain was gaining in intensity as we took to the sky. Initially, we could make out villages and towns below through gaps in the thick rain clouds. But the clouds soon closed ranks in an opaque barrier.

The cloud cover broke up after a while, revealing a reddish-brown expanse of bare earth that gradually gave way to a pastoral green. Then it emerged, in full view, its slopes adorned with a spiral of snow-white clouds, its legendary peak poking above the white adornment. Kilimanjaro!

Yohei, noting my excitement, urged our traveling companion, Nippon Foundation (then) executive director Tatsuya Tanami, to trade seats with me. Tanami graciously shifted to an open seat next to his window seat and ceded to me the perch with a view. I looked at a map and realized that our plane was heading south along the Great Rift Valley.

We began to see villages and the red-brown straight line of a road that cut through the forest. I watched expectantly for the appearance of Lake Malawi, but clouds again enveloped our aircraft as we began our descent to Lilongwe International Airport and robbed us of any such view.

Tough questions from the local press corps

A winter breeze offset the heat imparted by the bright sunlight at the airport in the 1,000-meter-plus-high Malawian capital. The bracing cool air was a welcome contrast with the summer swelter that we had left behind in Tokyo.

On hand to welcome Yohei were the director of the health ministry's preventive health unit, Dr. Storn Kabuluzi; the national professional officer at the WHO's Malawi office, Dr. Kelias Msyamboza; and the officer in charge of leprosy at the WHO's Republic of the Congo–based regional office for Africa, Dr. Landry Bide. The only discordant note to our arrival was the absence of 9 of the 10 bags that we had checked through to Lilongwe.

"That's rare," sighed Yohei. "For 2 or 3 bags to turn up missing is a common occurrence. But for nearly all the bags to miss the flight...!"

Yohei's face expressed his discomfiture, but he retained his characteristic grace. Nippon Foundation personnel quickly got in touch with the airline and determined where the bags were being held. They secured assurance from the airline that the bags would arrive the next day on a flight from Addis Ababa.

Our hosts escorted us through the airport building, a simple one-story affair, to a building next door. Awaiting us there were a television crew from a local station and three newspaper reporters. Yohei, calm and collected, addressed the impromptu press conference and its television audience with a localized version of the message that he delivers in nations worldwide.

"The Republic of Malawi has brought leprosy largely under control, thanks to excellent work by the Ministry of Health. A problem that remains is the discrimination that accompanies this disease. I am counting on the people of Malawi to move on from controlling leprosy to eliminating it completely. I call on you to realize that leprosy is not some kind of divine punishment, that it is not very contagious at all, and that prompt treatment with medicines can cure the disease.

"Viewers, please understand that leprosy is a purely medical problem. Please do not discriminate against the sufferers of the disease. I hold hands with them and hug them, and look: I don't have a trace of the disease. Please recognize sufferers as fellow human beings and treat them as fellow villagers.

"I am a Japanese and have traveled 32 hours to get here. Your nation and Japan have built good relations. Japan Overseas Cooperation Volunteers are active here. And I look forward to seeing our nations develop even closer ties."

The WHO standard for leprosy's elimination as a public health issue is less than 1 registered patient per 10,000 people. Malawi attained that standard overall in 1994, but 4 of the nation's 28 districts had yet to attain the standard at the time of our visit. Malawi had 321 new cases of leprosy in 2010, and the aggregate number of registered patients was equivalent to 0.5 per 10,000 people.

Yohei had received reports that cited four problems in the struggle to eradicate leprosy in Malawi. The first problem was the low priority assigned to leprosy in public health administration. That undermined accuracy in the gathering and transmission of patient data. The second problem was the lack of periodic visits to the districts by experts to provide guidance and supervision. The third problem was inadequate education for health workers in regard to leprosy. And the fourth problem was insufficient medium- and long-term planning for coordinating the fight against leprosy.

The litany of problems was daunting, and each of the four was attributable at least in part to a shortage of resources: human, financial, and material. Yohei was aware of the situation and had returned to Malawi after an 11-year hiatus to elicit a strengthened commitment from the government.

A female reporter in a dark-blue skirt emblazoned with a floral pattern brushed back her long curly hair and lobbed a question at Yohei. "How," she asked, "are we supposed to ensure that patients receive the treatment they need?"

"I travel the world in my fight against leprosy," began Yohei, "and I encounter places where people who have contracted leprosy don't know of their affliction or, even if they do, don't have access to physicians. Symptoms of the disease become visible, and the patients hide to avoid detection. So we need to go find the persons afflicted by the disease."

A male reporter in a shirt of dark-blue, white, and black stripes asked the next question. "Why do people discriminate against the sufferers of leprosy?"

"That's an excellent question," Yohei responded after giving the query some thought. "Humans have been discriminating against other humans since before the days of the Old Testament. I believe that discrimination began with leprosy."

The question was almost naïve in its directness. Malawi ranked near the bottom of the African rankings for annual gross national income per capita, at $290. Hand-to-mouth existence had perhaps instilled a cut-to-the-chase directness. And Yohei opted to respond in kind. He drew on the example of the Old Testament because he knew that about 75% of Malawians are Christian. That is a legacy of British colonial rule, which continued until 1964. Part and parcel of that legacy is English's standing as an official language alongside Chichewa.

"Leprosy can disfigure sufferers severely," Yohei continued. "People tend to want to keep disfigured members of society out of sight. That explains our history of exiling sufferers of leprosy to uninhabited islands and other remote settings. That happened in the Americas and in Europe, as well as in Africa. It also happened in my nation, Japan. We refused to respect the humanity of people who had contracted the disease.

"Today, leprosy has become a disease that is curable. Yet victims continue to experience discrimination even after they have recovered from the disease. They can't get jobs. They can't get married. They can't get on the bus. That sort of discrimination persists. My mission is to put an end to that discrimination."

"Why did you take up this work?" asked the female reporter.

"I accompanied my father on a visit to a leprosy colony in [the Republic of] Korea when I was 26. That was when I saw leprosy patients for the first time. Here were people that the world refused to acknowledge as human, and that realization hit me like a ton of bricks. I resolved then and there to do whatever I could to rid the world of leprosy, to rid the world of discrimination against the sufferers of the disease."

Thus ended the unscheduled press conference. We would visit a leprosy colony the next day, and I wondered why the reporters were coming after Yohei with questions now, before they had seen the facilities. I could see that they knew nothing about leprosy, but I suspected that their readers and viewers throughout the nation were equally ignorant of the disease. And I realized that Yohei's responses went right to the heart of what they ought to know about leprosy.

We got to our hotel at 6:30 p.m. It had the look of a resort, but a briefing by the Ministry of Health commenced before we had the chance to unwind. The minister was there when we arrived, but he had disappeared somewhere. A ministry official stood next to Yohei and read to him from a sheet of paper. As near as I could tell, he was going over a list of expenditures. Yohei was leaning over the sheet of paper and absorbing the explanation, but he ultimately raised his head, folded his arms, and turned his gaze away in a look of indignation.

The official seemed to be saying that he had no funds, no budget for combating leprosy. Malawi's government was apparently at a dead end in regard to measures for eradicating the disease. The shortage of funds was readily apparent at the ministry-hosted dinner that began at seven o'clock in the hotel ballroom. The minister, Professor David Mphande, had reappeared and delivered remarks in which he outlined the issue.

Malawi had some 350 new leprosy patients, lamented the minister, but a lot of them were far from clinics. Even basic motorcycles were unaffordable for numerous Malawians, he added, and commuting to the clinics was therefore impossible. The WHO's Bide, seated at the same table as me, shook his head as if to reject this explication.

"Awareness of leprosy is simply too low," Bide confided to me during the minister's talk. "The number of newly discovered patients is suspect. We can't trust the government reports. Leprosy is just about the lowest priority in health and sanitation here, and it receives practically no attention. To be sure, Malawi really had achieved the WHO's 'elimination' benchmark [of less than 1 case per 10,000 population] in 1994. But the government hasn't done anything since then about the disease."

I asked why things had slipped.

"Malawi is an extremely poor nation," Bide answered. "It relies on handouts from the United Kingdom. They could do better at managing things here. But it's landlocked and less accessible than most other African nations, so medical supplies don't arrive easily. We face serious geopolitical obstacles here."

"Most of the world's poorest one billion people have some kind of tropical disease," added Dr. Toshiyasu Shimizu, the officer in charge of tropical diseases at the WHO's regional office for Africa, who was sitting beside me across from Bide. "The diseases," he continued, "aren't necessarily fatal but can render the afflicted individuals blind or lame. I want to help those people, and I have proposed tackling leprosy along with tropical diseases, but Sasakawa-san doesn't show much sympathy for that approach."

Shimizu's comments revealed a vexing difficulty for those working to eradicate leprosy in Africa. The health ministries in all the sub-Saharan nations are working assiduously on measures for combating tropical diseases, but leprosy tends to get neglected in that prioritizing. Shimizu and like-minded individuals want to correct that omission by bundling leprosy with tropical diseases in survey work in Africa and Latin America.

Yohei's resistance to the bundled approach reflects his concern about the horrific discrimination that has historically accompanied leprosy. He regards eliminating that discrimination as a crucial facet of the battle against leprosy, and he worries that bundling leprosy with other diseases would leave that facet unaddressed. When Yohei's turn came to speak, he sounded as if he'd been eavesdropping on the conversation at our table. He began with a reference to the UN resolution that calls for ending discrimination against individuals affected by leprosy, and he continued in that vein.

"Malawi, the most beautiful nation on the African continent, has numerous people afflicted with such disorders as HIV, AIDS, and malaria. I am fully aware of that problem. But my principal concern is leprosy, and we have supported the Malawian government in the fight against that disease. I call on you to devote as much attention to leprosy as you do to tropical diseases. Leprosy has been the subject of loathing since before the time of the Old Testament. Its sufferers have experienced discrimination even after they have recovered from the disease. Lending our hands to the struggle to end that discrimination is a lofty calling for us as human beings."

A passion to end the discrimination experienced by a father

We left our hotel the next morning at eight o'clock and headed for the leprosy colony on our itinerary. The journalists overslept, so we set out in advance. Waiting would have meant not reaching our destination until after noon. I had learned quickly that Malawians are not especially preoccupied with punctuality.

Our hotel stood amid lovely verdure atop a well-kept rise. We soon encountered something of a traffic jam where vehicles were lined up at the only gasoline station in the vicinity. But the police jeep that was escorting us to the leprosy colony turned on its siren and light and cut a path for us through the congestion. Police officers also sat in the front passenger seat and in the bed of our four-wheel-drive vehicle, but they were unarmed. Malawi has been free of civil war and coups d'état since independence, and it is a generally safe and peaceful nation.

We were out of central Lilongwe in no time at all. Even in the city center, nary a high-rise building was to be seen. The only architecture of note was a complex of stately, low-rise government buildings on a gently sloping tract of land. And immediately after leaving the city, we passed villages that were right out of the movies. Our road was paved, but the asphalt was little more than a thin carpet lain directly on the red earth. I had the feeling that I could have peeled it away with one hand. Unpaved red lanes ran left and right from the road to forest villages.

Soon, we left the forest behind and entered a long stretch of alternating fields and woods. Small houses lined the road. Some were of brick, but most were simple mud-and-straw huts with thatched roofs. They bore the black soot of the fireplaces inside, and above each rose a plume of smoke.

"People in houses like those keep fires burning around the clock," noted Yohei while looking out the window. "The fires keep the bugs at bay. Cutting wood for the fires destroys the forests. The development agency of another African nation sought to protect the trees by teaching the people to use charcoal. But that only made things worse. Do you know why?"

Yohei continued without waiting for an answer and without taking his eyes off the scenery passing by outside the window.

"It's a remarkable story. People wanted the charcoal, and they needed money to buy it, so they cut down more trees to get the money."

"Just another case," I nodded, "of well-intentioned initiatives going awry."

"Africa's a difficult place to make improvements in patterns of behavior," Yohei observed. "Europeans made a mess of things here. They ruled by setting the tribes against each other, giving them guns and ammunition and money. The Europeans then made off with the resources."

That prompted me to ask about something that had been on my mind since we arrived in Malawi.

"You talked about discrimination in fielding questions from the reporters at the airport yesterday. But I wonder if they even really understand what you mean by that word. Could you please tell me more about how the issue of discrimination figures in your fight against leprosy?"

"What drives me," said Yohei emphatically, "is anger at discrimination. My work is, at root, a fight against discrimination."

I waited silently for Yohei to continue, which he did, turning from the window to look me in the eye.

"My running around the world like this in the fight against leprosy and against discrimination stems from an ever-so-serious motivation. I want to dispel the discrimination that my father experienced. He was a prominent right-wing figure [before, during, and after the war], and the occupation forces arrested him as a suspected Class A war criminal, though they released him without bringing formal charges. The media in Japan have branded him as a gambling racketeer who funneled his ill-gotten gains into charitable works.

"I urged my father I don't know how many times to sue the media for defamation of character. But he'd always tell me, 'Hey, the reporters writing that stuff have got to eat, too. They've got to care for their families. Still, I don't like the way that their slander spawns misunderstanding even beyond Japan, and I'd like to set things straight.'"

Scorched-earth evidence of slash-and-burn agriculture came into view. So did a village of low dwellings.

"People associated [my father] with wrongdoing and with violence," Yohei went on. "They spoke of him in the same breath with [the notorious racketeer] Yoshio Kodama [1911–1984]. I spent seven years getting my father's materials in order and then turned them over to the University of Tokyo historian Takashi Ito [1932–]. We archived the materials in five volumes, and Ito-san wrote a one-volume biography. Read those books, and you will see clearly that the accusations against my father are utterly unfounded. My father, by the way, never felt victimized in the least. Next July 18 is the 16th anniversary of his death. When we've got past that milestone [the 17th anniversary in the Japanese counting system], I'll be free to concentrate on my own affairs."

I'd heard from Yohei in Tokyo about his perceptions of discrimination against his father. But this was the first time I'd heard about him spending seven years compiling an archival and biographical record. I was amazed at how far he'd gone in acting on his filial instincts. Takashi Ito was a prominent historian, famed especially for unearthing a wealth of primary materials that illuminate recent Japanese history. A remarkable sense of commitment was evident in Yohei's readiness to present such an authority with primary materials about Ryoichi Sasakawa and to seek an honest appraisal.

"Are you seeking revenge?" I caught myself even as the words were leaving my mouth. A vengeful motivation would, of course, be unrelenting. If we attribute lofty, universal goals and actions in their pursuit to a fundamental drive rooted in the individual, we can attribute Yohei's work to personal passion. And that grand work, driven by passion, conveys a message far more powerful than anything of purely intellectual grounding.

We passed by a marketplace. Peaks loomed in the foreground. We had ascended into high country and were entering the mountains. The red earth climbed ever upward. Our road had long since lost any semblance of pavement, and our vehicle rocked every which way on the bumpy terrain. The ride tossed Yohei about as if he was on a trampoline.

"I call this a massage chair," Yohei laughed. "And it twists your bowels as part of the bargain."

Children carrying firewood on their heads walked alongside the road. We also saw adults carrying full-to-the-brim water buckets on their heads and the elderly carrying stalks of sugarcane longer than themselves on their heads. All were wearing T-shirts and walking barefoot. The stream of people of all ages carrying daily essentials on their heads went on seemingly forever.

The vegetation around us turned a darker shade of green. A river was visible through the trees. Soon, we came out into a village. Children waved.

"Do you suppose these people give any thought to death?" I pondered aloud.

"They accept their fate," stated Yohei with conviction. "These people will amaze you. Japanese flounder about with the fear of death, and some even kill themselves. These villagers are incredible. The villagers experience joy and sadness. They rise with the sun and go to bed when the sun goes down. People in rich countries say that we've got to do something about the poverty in Africa, but they can't solve the problem. I just want to do what I can in the way of medical care."

My watch showed 9:45 a.m. We had arrived at the top of a mountain, or so I thought. In fact, we were crossing a pass. The road turned gradually downward. We came into another village. Again, the children waved. Electric poles, which we hadn't seen earlier, supplied the village with power. I'd been concerned on hearing that electrification reached only about 10% of the territory in Malawi. On the other hand, I noted enviously the absence of advertising billboards. I marveled at the freedom and at the unadulterated human interaction that would prevail in a world free of incessant pressure to "buy, buy."

"Take a look along the sides of the road," urged Yohei. "You don't see trash piled up anywhere, and we haven't seen any the whole way. I guess the stuff gets recycled here. Nigeria was horrible. Vinyl garbage was flying around everywhere. Here, everyone seems to keep things tidy."

Yohei then turned silent. I sensed that he was stuck on something, and I offered an observation to get him started again.

"On the other hand, it might be that the people here simply don't have things to be throwing away."

"Saving face is important in poor nations," Yohei resumed. "The places that my hosts show me are presumably the better side of things. That's something that I can understand."

With that, Yohei closed his eyes. We'd experienced something similar in Mumbai. Only by asking children could you get honest answers about the lives of the elderly. I didn't think that people had picked up trash in advance of our visit on government orders. But I did remind myself to be a rigorous observer of whatever awaited us at the leprosy colony ahead.

"They say that the health minister here is caring for 25 family members," said Yohei. "He's lost two brothers and has taken their families under his wing.

Even a government minister is abiding by the African tradition of tending a large family. The familial bonds are strong here."

Yohei turned his reopened eyes to me and continued.

"Confucius's teachings of 2,500 years ago are as valid as ever today. We humans haven't changed a bit over the past two-and-a-half millennia. A lion lies sprawled on the savanna, and a zebra walks by utterly unafraid. Why? Because the zebra knows that the lion is full, knows that the lion is content with what's enough. People don't understand what's enough without being told. Some don't understand even when they are told. But this comes instinctively to animals in nature. And our leaders go on pretentiously about gathering for summits. Do you know about Tanzania's Ngorongoro Conservation Area?"

I shook my head.

"A volcanic eruption left a huge crater, and different kinds of big animals live there: lions, elephants, rhinoceroses, hippopotamuses, wildebeests, even zebras, which are prey for lions. The crater is also home to lots of birds and smaller animals. Maasai long raised cattle there, too. The ecosystem maintained that diversity perfectly well. Then the World Economic Forum goes and holds an African economic summit there. We ought to give some thought to how our lifestyles have deteriorated amid diversity, to how scientific and technological progress has warped our lives."

Yohei possesses an encyclopedic mind. He can summon a cartographic perspective on the world at any time, can cite the ethnic groups and the political leaders in each nation, can discourse at length on the history of civilization in each nation and region. I've heard from Yohei that he was never much of a reader until his was 60. But in the past decade, he's achieved an impressive erudition that spans East and West. That he has been able to do that is testimony to a character that is young at heart. It is also testimony to an immunity from prideful rigidity and to a readiness to discard preconceptions and attachments one after another.

What has shaped Yohei's perspective most definitively, however, has been his on-the-ground experience of remote precincts around the world. Leprosy is more prevalent in undeveloped areas than in urban areas, and the people in those areas tend to be economically poor and dependent on the natural bounty of their immediate environment. Yohei accompanies book learning with the direct experience of having shared tears and laughter with peoples left behind by progress, left to a premodern mode of life.

The person who awakened Yohei to the joy of reading was Keiichi Torii, a special adviser (now a counselor) at the Nippon Foundation. Torii came to the foundation from Fuji Television Network, Inc., where he had covered political affairs and served as the Saigon (now Ho Chi Minh City) bureau chief during the Vietnam War. When Yohei sought to compile his father's papers for publishing, Torii introduced Takashi Ito as a suitable editor and writer. Torii was also responsible for persuading another University of Tokyo professor, the political scientist Seisaburo Sato (1932–1999), to write a book about Yohei's father: *Sasakawa Ryoichi kenkyu: Ijigen kara no shisha* (A Study of Ryoichi Sasakawa: a messenger from another dimension [Tokyo: Chuokoron-sha, Inc., 1998]).

Torii would make book recommendations, and Yohei would read the books faithfully, cover to cover, like a good student. Yohei used the time on planes, in airports, and elsewhere to read books, and the books he read were invariably those recommended by Torii.

Our vehicle lurched upward. Yohei's eyes were closed. Outside the window was the pacific scene of a village and more scorched earth of slash-and-burn cultivation. Low green cover had taken hold on the dry soil. At first glance, I thought of soybeans, but a closer look revealed the telltale white wisps of cotton plants. Punctuating the scene were miniature Towers of Babel— anthills I had known only from photographs. As the greenery swayed in the breeze, a group of children, perhaps three or four years old, approached. Eyes that flashed like crystal looked us over.

Three immense baobab trees of unworldly configuration stood at the edge of the forest. I recalled the distinctive baobab tree that we had seen at a leprosarium in Egypt and mulled over the arboreal distinctions occasioned by different climes. The trunks of these specimens were bulbous, like beer kegs, their bark smooth to the eye. Short branches, adorned with leaves, projected out like sparklers. I speculated about how the French post-impressionist Henri Rousseau (1844–1910) would have rendered the comically mysterious form of the baobab.

As much dead as alive

More than three hours after leaving our hotel, we arrived at the leprosy colony. Emblazoned on the gate was the enigmatic indication "Father's House," though Utale was the facility's formal name. We had traveled 230 kilometers southeast from Lilongwe to the parched terrain of the Balaka District. That smallish district has a population of about 340,000, including 31 registered leprosy patients. Its prevalence of 0.9 patients per 10,000 residents is a little higher than the average for Malawi overall.

French Catholic missionaries settled in what is now the Balaka District in the 1920s, and they established the Utale colony in 1946 as an isolation sanatorium for leprosy patients. The missionaries established five leprosy colonies in Malawi, but the Utale facility, we heard, is the only one of theirs that remains. It housed 34 patients and former patients in an on-site rehabilitation center at the time of our visit, and 43 cured persons had moved to a nearby village.

The colony remained under the administration of Catholic missionaries, led by the priest Francis Kachere. Our guide was the medical director. We soon saw in the clinic that the facility accommodated outpatients for ailments other than leprosy. The outpatients received treatment in a small room reached through a narrow passage. Multidrug therapy blister packs were in storage on shelves.

"You need to sign in," the director instructed us brusquely at the pristine reception desk. "We wash their feet here so that they won't transmit diseases."

I was surprised at what awaited us on the grounds of the rehabilitation center. Dwellings stood in neat rows and presented an appearance more beautiful than any of the villages that we had passed on the way. More than a snapshot of poverty-stricken life, this was a picturesque village scene that anyone would find appealing. The main street through the village carried hardly any vehicular traffic, and rows of trees provided shade on both sides of the street. Lining the sidewalks were brick sheds of a bright color scheme that lent a sense of warmth to the setting. The director told us that they were the work of Father Kachere and the other missionaries. People had wandered out onto the sidewalks for the sun.

"They are former patients," explained the director in a calm and reassuring voice. "All of them live here."

"This is almost too good to be true," exuded Yohei with a big and ingratiating smile.

We encountered some modest entrepreneurship as we began walking. A man who looked to be in his 60s had brought out a sewing machine and was engaged in seamstering for the other residents. He displayed no conspicuous aftereffects of leprosy on his face or limbs. Yohei sat down beside the tailor and said encouragingly, "You're doing great. God is with you."

"He received early treatment," commented the director. "That's why he's in such good shape."

We next came upon a woman who also appeared to be 60 something and who was sitting directly on the sidewalk. She plucked bits of leaf from a cigarette, stuffed them in both her nostrils, and inhaled hard. The woman presented Yohei with some pluckings from the cigarette and challenged him to have a go. He took her up on the challenge but choked on the leaf and sneezed, eliciting laughter. I also got into the act but was unable to enjoy that sort of smokeless snuff. All that I got from the experience was a stinging in my nasal passages.

Yohei stopped at each dwelling. Lounging in front of one was a young man. He reported that he had a wife and six children. He exhibited no signs of leprosy.

"You detected your disease early on, didn't you?" asked Yohei.

"I got medicine and was cured in six months."

"How did you learn that you had the disease."

"The doctor here discovered it when I came for treatment for another problem."

"That's fantastic."

Yohei shook the young man's hand, and we moved on. You would think that people who had been cured of the disease would move back to their home villages. That they had chosen to remain in Utale was evidence that going home was not an option. The young man's wife and six children were nowhere to be seen, which made me wonder what sort of living arrangements the family had made.

Sadly, the aftereffects of leprosy were more than evident in most of the older residents. Yohei sat down between two elderly women. The woman on his left was wearing a blank expression and was holding her cadaverous cheeks in her hands. Gaping cracks in the skin of her deformed legs were attracting clusters of flies. Yohei brushed away the flies as he struck up a conversation.

"I don't know if I'm dead or alive," muttered the woman in a feeble voice. Yohei grasped one of her fingerless hands and wrapped his free arm around her shoulders. Her face, framed in a scarf, was that of a witch who had been robbed of her magical powers.

"Where are you from?" asked Yohei.

"I'm from Mozambique. My family threw me out when I got this disease. I couldn't even stay in my village, so I came here on my own."

Yohei's face wrinkled as he offered encouragement to the woman.

"God is looking after you. This is a wonderful village. God's guidance has brought you here."

Yohei was not a person who commonly spoke of God or of God's guidance. However, the woman and all the residents here were presumably Christian, and Yohei had employed language that they would understand. He next turned to the woman on his right, but his greeting elicited not so much as a flick of her glance.

"She can't hear," said the woman from Mozambique. She apparently couldn't speak either. Yohei stared intently into her face. Her eyes were as lacking in life as those of the men we had met at the leprosarium in Alexandria. "Ah, this person's eyesight is gone," Yohei concluded.

A youngish-looking man who was sitting nearby and dressed in deep blue had his eyes open, but they were as white as milk. He got up, supporting his gaunt frame unsteadily with a white cane. He was dragging his right leg awkwardly, and a man of large build noticed and came over to help. They held opposite ends of the cane and walked off somewhere like children playing train. The sight made me wonder if, even here, people didn't avoid direct contact with the visibly afflicted.

Lots of people who had all manner of deformities had come out and were sitting or walking along the street. The entrepreneurs hawked their goods. The sky was a cloudless and flawless blue. Yet a quiet enveloped the tableau that was simply eerie, garnished only by occasional flecks of windborne sand. A biblical verse came to mind. "Yea, though I walk through the valley of the shadow of death, I will fear no evil: for thou art with me; thy rod and thy staff they comfort me" (Psalm 23:4 [King James Version]).

The notion of human fraternity

We found the congregation hall on another street. Yohei entered through an open door. Resounding from within were the voices of women singing. The men didn't sing here. When the choral harmony was over, we again heard the turkey-gobble trilling that we had heard in Egypt. This welcome, I realized, was not unique to the Arab world.

The sleepyhead journalists chose this timing to make their appearance. Residents and visitors alike crowded into the not especially spacious congregation hall. A tall, thin, and broad-shouldered man was making some sort of greeting to Yohei. Laughter arose occasionally from the female contingent. The people seated in the rows from the middle to the front of the gathering sat on the floor, their legs jutting forward. From the middle to the back of the hall, people sat in chairs.

A flock of ducks proceeded down the street in front of the hall, and the cacophonous quacking rendered the man's voice difficult to discern. The noisy ducks had passed slowly down the street when the director's turn came to speak. He went on forever, reciting a long list of shortages and requests for assistance.

While the director was talking, I viewed the legs of the women in the front rows. I marveled at how the women could sit with their legs extended like that through the interminable talk. And as I gradually made out the dark-skinned limbs in the dim light, I realized that all of them were hideously disfigured. Some of the legs were toeless and had swollen to elephantine proportions, the nerves presumably long dead. Some of the women suffered additionally from blindness.

Yohei's turn came to speak.

"Thank you for turning out like this and for your gracious welcome. I regard the world as one big house and all the people of the world as parents, as sisters, as brothers. Today, I have come a long way to be here, and I am extremely happy at this chance to meet with my brothers and sisters."

The wording was a borrowing from phraseology familiar to Japanese from the public-interest TV commercials run by Yohei's father, Ryoichi Sasakawa: "Humankind is one family. All human beings all brothers." This was the first time I had heard Yohei utter those words. I could see, more than ever, that Yohei revered his father and was committed to carrying on in his father's spirit.

"For people to experience discrimination because they have contracted leprosy," Yohei continued, "makes no sense. The people who suffer discrimination have done nothing wrong. The people who discriminate are doing something very wrong. [Applause.] By no means is this disease divine punishment for anything. It is just a disease, like tuberculosis and malaria. I shook hands with a lot of you here today. And I have had contact with countless leprosy patients and former patients over the decades that I have been doing this work. But look. I have never contracted the disease. The ordinary people who live in Malawi have wrong notions about leprosy, and that's wrong. Most of you are also citizens of Malawi. You have exactly the same rights as the other citizens."

Uncharacteristically, Yohei had not referred to the UN resolution that calls for eliminating discrimination against people afflicted directly or indirectly by leprosy. He usually cited that resolution in his remarks to gatherings like the one here. I assumed that he was tailoring his remarks to the educational level of the audience.

Yohei announced that he was presenting the colony with a gift of €800 and invited everyone able to join him in a dance. Cheerful music played, and those able to stand got up and danced and sang. The dancing and singing continued for two numbers, and that brought the gathering to an end.

"Meeting people like that always leaves me with mixed emotions," acknowledged Yohei on the way back to the hotel. He looked a little fatigued. "Why wasn't I born in this country? Why wasn't I born as one of those people? I could well have been one of those people. When you think of it like that, you could regard them as having shouldered my fate in my place. That reinforces my sense of mission in carrying out this work. I get that feeling every time I come away from an on-site visit. This was the first time that officials from the health ministry had visited a leprosy colony. That's a reminder that I need to keep up my efforts."

The police in the escort jeep that we were trailing turned on their siren. That was a warning to our driver to be wary of the potholes in the road. The jeep bobbed up and down, and we did likewise. We were barreling along at 120 kilometers per hour over a road where half that speed would have seemed excessive.

"From now on," Yohei continued, "little strokes will overcome big folks. That has to happen. Ordinary people who have been dominated by politics will turn the tables and dominate politics. At the very least, corporations need to fulfill their social responsibility. I've got three slogans in mind: Share the pain. Share the hope. And share the future. I want to position those as guiding themes for the foundation. I haven't yet mentioned this to anyone on the staff, though."

Yohei turned his gaze to the passing scenery outside the window.

Inspiring remarks and a chilling realization

Our hotel in Lilongwe was comfortable. Each room had a terrace that overlooked a courtyard. The day after our excursion to Utale, we breakfasted at six thirty on our terraces, coddled by a cool breeze. The only thing on Yohei's schedule that day was a late-afternoon joint press conference with the minister of health. We had decided to use our free time to go see Lake Malawi.

When I met Yohei at the hotel entrance at seven thirty, the WHO's Bide had been lecturing him intently about something. Yohei turned to me with an atypically troubled look.

"The Ministry of Health is hiding things," he murmured. "When I asked to visit a hospital, they told me that the hospitals were closed today. Meanwhile, I've discovered that Malawi has more than one leprosy colony. Nonprofit organizations are running colonies besides the Utale facility. My guess is that the others are in pretty bad shape. Catholic missionaries run the Utale colony, so it's in pretty good shape. It's one of the best-run colonies that I've seen anywhere."

Yohei wasn't suggesting that the Ministry of Health was violating accepted norms to conceal its policy shortcomings. Rather, he was noting that it was conforming with accepted norms in sub-Saharan Africa. He knew the "givens," and he wanted to find a way to overcome them and achieve his goal here at the wrong end of the poverty spectrum. His goal, of course, was to raise awareness in Malawi about the need for eradicating leprosy and for eradicating discrimination against those affected by the disease. And achieving that goal would mean persuading those in power to devote heightened priority to the cause.

Getting to Lake Malawi would take, we'd heard, about three hours, so we'd need to turn back almost as soon as we got there. Yohei welcomed the jaunt nonetheless as an opportunity for viewing the lives of people along the way.

Off we went on another red-earth road, rambling along between slash-and-burn aftermath and cotton fields. We encountered no other vehicles, and our driver explained that the bicycle is the luxury vehicle of Malawi. Children walked empty handed along the side of the road. In time, the villages that had popped into view intermittently stopped appearing altogether, and our road narrowed as we found ourselves traversing a forest.

A baby elephant emerged from the sylvan shadow and cut across the road before our eyes. We reached the edge of the lake at 10:15. The lake seemed as vast as an ocean. Standing beside an inlet, we observed three parent-and-child pairs of hippopotamuses on the other side of the water. That view, along with a close-up view of dried hippopotamus droppings that would have made excellent fertilizer, was our souvenir of Lake Malawi.

"The president doesn't seem to want to see us," grumbled Yohei when we were in the vehicle and back on the road. "I'm following up through our contact, but we supposedly had a commitment to meet."

A curious form that was wiggling on a sloping field outside had captured my eye. It appeared to be human, but it was legless and was pulling itself up the slope, insect like, with both arms. I could only speculate as to what sort of disability the person, if it was indeed a person, had, and what her or his purpose was in climbing the slope. I prayed that he or she was not someone suffering from the aftereffects of leprosy. But I knew that numerous such individuals went without care in this nation and had to make their way through life as best they could.

Yohei's joint press conference with the minister of health got under way at 3:20. It took place in a meeting room in the white, modern building that housed the ministry atop a gentle rise. Yohei, as always, called for correcting misconceptions about leprosy. He emphasized that medicine for treating the disease was available free of charge from the Malawian government and that leprosy, if detected early, could be cured completely without leaving any aftereffects. Yohei also repeated his lamentation about discrimination persisting even after people had been cured of the disease. And he noted the unanimous ratification of the UN resolution that calls for ending discrimination against people affected by leprosy.

"I made this visit to Malawi," Yohei explained, "because of an increase, albeit small, in the incidence of leprosy here. The Ministry of Health has succeeded in achieving the elimination of leprosy as a public health problem, and I am counting on the government to raise the priority that it devotes to eradicating the disease. I visited the Utale facility yesterday and heard the requests of the people there. The district commissioner was there, and I learned that his office is compiling a list of requests of patients and former patients and of their family members. This visit has reinforced my confidence in the potential for eradicating leprosy in your nation. And I am grateful to the minister of health for the gracious invitation to be here."

Mphande, the health minister, applauded Yohei's remarks heartily. A large-framed man of 72, he could well have passed for 50-something and was wearing a well-tailored, dark-blue suit. I knew that he must be a capable and generous individual to be caring for 25 family members, and his remarks, straightforward and sincere, reinforced that impression. He described how the prevalence of leprosy in Malawi had declined from 0.57 per 10,000 people in 2008 to 0.45 in 2009 but had edged up to 0.5 in 2010. "I don't know why," he acknowledged frankly about the uptick.

Yohei's visit was prompting Mphande to rethink fundamentally his ministry's approach to leprosy. The minister had first met Yohei at the WHO's World Health Assembly in Geneva in May 2010. When Yohei asked at that time about visiting Malawi, Mphande exhibited no awareness of the leprosy problem in his nation.

"I will fight to bring the prevalence of leprosy here down to zero," declared Mphande in front of the television cameras. "The Republic of Malawi will rise to this challenge. Let us achieve the total elimination of leprosy in our nation. I am grateful to Sasakawa-san, who has come to promote that quest. We will eliminate leprosy. We will eradicate the disease. We will fight to achieve that goal. That is my pledge. This disease is curable. I call on you in the media to convey that message to our citizens."

Yohei rose while clapping and shook hands with the minister. Mphande had impressed me with his obvious sense of commitment. Next came tough questions from the media.

"How can you talk of eradication when we still have patients here?"

"The prevalence is 0.5 per 10,000 people in 2010," replied a ministry official. "So we speak of zero [in the sense of having brought the disease under control]. But we realize that we still have citizens who have the disease."

"We still have a few patients," added Mphande. "But even former patients suffer discrimination. We need to cure the patients, and we need to allow those who have been cured to return to society. That means eliminating discrimination."

Some 15 or 16 journalists were on hand for the press conference, and hands shot up next from 4 of them at once. The moderator called on all 4 as a group.

"Does your zero target mean that you will increase the number of facilities?"

"How long will getting to zero take?"

"How many patients are at Utale?"

"Utale isn't the only facility, is it? We have other leprosy colonies, don't we?"

The last of the questions was from a female journalist, and her query, delivered in a pleasant but uncompromising tone, put the ministry officials on the spot. The official who fielded the questions handled them as a bundle. He didn't say whether the ministry would increase the number of facilities or offer a time line for reducing the prevalence to zero.

As for existing facilities, "leprosy colonies operate in Machinga, in Balaka, and in Mchinji, as well as in Utale," the official acknowledged. "We will begin monitoring all of the facilities rigorously. We have facilities in a total of eight districts."

The ministry had no precise information about the facilities because it had neglected them completely. Mphande, who seemed determined to address all the queries fully, rose again.

"We still have leprosy in the Republic of Malawi," the minister acknowledged. "The Ministry of Health will fight to eradicate the disease. A strong partner has appeared in the form of Sasakawa-san. We will tackle this fight with Sasakawa-san. I look forward to the day when we can announce that we have eradicated leprosy."

I found the remarks by Mphande genuinely inspiring. And while I was feeling inspired, my eyes lit on something that gave me a chill. Hanging on the wall was something utterly un-Malawian: a hanging scroll from China. The shadow of Chinese influence was darkening by the day over this nation.

Malawi had retained diplomatic ties with Taiwan until 2007. It cut those ties in that year, however, and established diplomatic relations with China. The Malawian government did not disclose details of any quid pro quo for switching its diplomatic allegiance, but China announced that it would provide Malawi with $260 million in concessionary loans, grants, and aid over five years. And that largesse was ongoing as we visited.

The scenery that we saw on the road in Malawi had included more than the villages, fields, and forests that I have described. Also in evidence were conspicuous examples of China's waxing influence. An immense, Chinese-funded stadium was under construction, for example, in the heart of Lilongwe. Visible at the construction site was a huge statue suggestive of a stern-looking god of victory. Sure enough, the sculptural style betrayed the statue's Middle Kingdom origins.

Also under construction in Lilongwe with Chinese financing were a new home for the National Assembly, a new official residence for the president, and an eight-story five-star hotel slated to include an international conference center. Plans were under way, too, for luxury villas in Lilongwe to be financed by Chinese sources. And China was preparing to help build a university of science and technology in southern Malawi.

I shuddered at the thought of the warm and endearing spirit of Africa succumbing to Chinese domination. The Chinese builders of the National Assembly building and the presidential residence could well install hidden cameras. They would thus gain a real-time window on the secret proceedings of high-level meetings and on illicit behavior whose propagators they could subject to extortion. The "beneficiaries" of the Chinese largesse will presumably be dependent on Chinese expertise for managing the computer system, the electric power supply, and other crucial functions.

None of the journalists at the press conference asked how the government would pay for the stepped-up eradication effort. Fully aware of the government's fiscal strictures, they might well have been steering clear of a sensitive subject intentionally.

Malawi's economic insignificance is apparent in the paucity of diplomatic missions in the nation. A staff member from the Japanese embassy who was at the press conference reported that the only Western missions there were the embassies of Germany, Iceland, Ireland, Norway, the United Kingdom, and the United States and the delegation of the European Union. Even the African diplomatic contingent was thin, consisting of the embassies of the neighboring nations of Mozambique, Tanzania, and Zambia and those of Egypt, South Africa, and Zimbabwe. Japan had only opened its embassy in 2008, and not a single Japanese parliamentarian had visited the nation in an official capacity.

Natural resources were sparse in Malawi, and the nation depended on tobacco for about 60% of its foreign exchange earnings. Small cultivators accounted for nearly all of the tobacco production, and prices were weakening on the global market amid the antismoking pressures that were mounting worldwide.

Fuel was an especially pressing issue for Malawians. Diesel was the overwhelmingly predominant source of mechanical power, and Malawi was short of cash resources for purchasing diesel fuel. That shortage impeded progress in addressing different development priorities, including the need for diversifying agricultural output. The government was encouraging farmers to shift to the production of coffee and cotton, but that shift hinged on access to diesel power for farm equipment.

Fines for flatulence

The day arrived, July 16, for our departure from Malawi. We needed to head for the airport soon after noon. The president had canceled his appointment with Yohei, who was philosophical. We would take the opportunity to visit the marketplace instead.

Our driver, short and thin, looked to be only around 20 years old, and he had decked himself out in a bright-red double-breasted suit. He had apparently borrowed the suit from a friend, someone considerably larger than himself, for today's work. The shoulders of the jacket drooped, the sleeves concealed the driver's hands, and the pant cuffs were folded neatly up inside the legs. Perched atop a thin neck, the smallish, close-shaved head could have been something that grew out of Malawi's red soil. The driver's innocently infectious smile flashed orderly rows of bright white teeth.

Lilongwe's marketplace sprawled over a hill in the old city center. A river flowed nearby. The vegetables on offer included green beans and all manner of other beans, ginger, tomatoes, round red chilies, and green peppers. Beyond the vegetables were rows of dried fish for sale. The narrow passageways cut a curving maze through the marketplace, diverging and converging, swelling and tightening. We saw no litter anywhere on the spotless grounds, and the fish stalls were totally free of flies.

Impinging on the mood were the menacing glares directed at us by men and women. The reason for the ill will became clear in vocal alarm, "Chinese!" To be sure, the speaker was not addressing us directly but, rather, announcing our presence to his colleagues. We could hear the news echoing on ahead, however, and we felt distinctly uncomfortable.

"Chinese are unpopular in Malawi," explained our driver and guide. "They build stadiums and hotels, but the Malawians who work in the projects get low wages. And they get slugged and kicked."

"This could get dangerous if we stay too long," added the driver in a low voice. We sensed that the driver's safety was at risk, too, and Yohei suggested that we leave. Open-air stalls on the other side of the river beckoned. I bought a wooden carving of mother-and-child elephants for the equivalent of about eight dollars. Back in the car, Yohei asked the driver about something funny that he'd heard.

"I heard that the president has proposed a law that would impose fines for farting. Is that true?"

"Yes, it's true," answered the ever-knowledgeable driver. "But the bill ran into opposition in the National Assembly and didn't pass. They have a law like that next door in Zambia."

"*Hey*, how about that," Yohei mused, punning on a Japanese word for "fart."

"The bill was supposed to be a measure for protecting the environment. People could have been arrested, as well as fined. But everybody farts, don't they? You'd have to arrest everyone in the country. You wouldn't have any people left. So the members of the National Assembly opposed the bill."

"How would you know that someone had farted? If it didn't happen right in front of a police officer, making an arrest would be impossible."

"No, you could report someone for farting and get them arrested."

"*Hey*, that's incredible. In that case, the citizens should have all turned themselves in. 'I farted, so arrest me.' They should have pulled that on the president."

Yohei was doing his best to keep from laughing. The driver started the car.

"The current president," the driver complained, "loves to find excuses to charge fines and raise taxes. Everyone is disgusted. Did you see the train line? The trains aren't running now. The previous president ran a trucking company, so he prohibited rail transport and forced everyone to switch to trucks. Now, the current president wants to restart rail transport. He wants to build a train line from Mozambique to Malawi."

A Brazilian company that has close ties with Mozambique is reportedly in on the president's proposed rail project, and Chinese companies would presumably get in on laying the tracks in Malawi. Presidents of poor countries put in place ludicrous laws to squeeze money out of ordinary people. Big countries take advantage. Malawi's average monthly income per capita was less than the equivalent of $100 a month at the time of our visit. Some 75% of the people were subsisting on less than the equivalent of a dollar a day. We were amazed to hear from our driver that he made only about $100 a year."

With us in the car was the Nippon Foundation's Tanami. As we headed for the airport, he shared some information about Malawi that he'd gleaned from the local newspaper and from some reporters.

"The Malawian government," reported Tanami, "has suffered one failure after another in political and economic undertakings. Medicine is in short supply, even in the hospitals. We're leaving this country today, but big antigovernment demonstrations will take place on the 20th, four days from now. I've learned that they'll take place all across the country, not just here in Lilongwe. The president has dismissed the vice president, a woman, and she's moving to form a new party. She and her supporters will take part in the antigovernment demonstrations in an effort to bring down the president. The president, meanwhile, is planning to give a speech at a rally on the same day to counter the opposition. Let's just hope that no bloodshed occurs."

We had heard repeatedly about the "peaceful African spirit." But keeping things peaceful had become all but impossible.

"This nation depends on foreign assistance for 40% of its economy," continued Tanami. "About half of the assistance is from the United Kingdom. The UK government has announced that it will terminate its assistance. That's why the government here is moving to raise taxes. That would impose a heavy burden on people like our driver."

I suspected that the driver would take part in an antigovernment demonstration. Changing the subject, I asked Yohei for his takeaways from our visit.

"I didn't say anything critical of the government at the press conference yesterday, did I?" he answered. "Criticizing poor countries is never in order." He folded his arms and continued. "I said that this nation could get the number of leprosy patients down to zero. The health minister responded by pledging to the nation's people to make that happen. Now, the government needs to make good on that pledge. Ideally, I'd like to have met with the president and to have secured the same pledge from him.

"AIDS and HIV patients outnumber leprosy patients here by two orders of magnitude. Numerically, leprosy is just an afterthought. That's why I wanted to get the president to order his people to devote some attention to this problem, too. I didn't get to meet with the president, but my visit generated some results nonetheless.

"Dr. Bide and others from the WHO will come here and work with the health ministry. They'll do survey work to see if any cases have gone undetected and to see if former patients are receiving the support that they require. Most important of all, the health ministry now has a commitment to eradicating leprosy that it needs to fulfill. The people at the WHO's regional office have been overly deferential toward their governmental counterparts in each nation. My visit prompted the health minister to speak passionately of 'fighting' to eradicate leprosy. The groundwork is now in place for a stepped-up effort."

A large photograph of the president's wedding hung on the wall along the route to the VIP lounge at the airport. I stopped and peered in amazement at the scene in the photo. He had staged an extravagant ceremony before thousands of guests in some sort of arena. The president was 77 years old, and he had gotten married when he was 72. His bride was 47 years old and was the minister of the environment at the time of the marriage. A comment in the car by our driver came to mind.

"Everyone says that he changed a lot after he got married. That's happens, I guess, if you marry someone 30 years younger."

The photograph of the bride and groom was simply unbelievable. I had no idea who they had commissioned to design their wedding garb. The worry-free smiles, however, were plainly bizarre. I could half imagine that someone had hung this photo here to undercut the reputation of the president. A more likely interpretation was that the president, insane with power, had commanded the hanging of the photo out of vanity.

I couldn't help suspecting that Chinese money had financed the ceremony. That would suggest that the president had sold out to the Chinese, a sin worse than outlawing flatulence. Rather than opposing the bill, the members of the National Assembly should have passed it and promptly had the president arrested for farting.

I turned to the WHO's Bide and asked, "Do you think that [Yohei's] visit was worthwhile?"

"Yes," Bide replied. "Getting things done will be a lot easier now. We've agreed on a schedule for doing the survey work. We'll do it this October. We'll travel with consultants to sites across the country. Representatives of the Malawi health ministry will come along too."

"Chairman Sasakawa has also expressed satisfaction with the visit."

"Formerly, people simply tossed ideas around. 'Let's do this. Let's do that.' But nothing got done. Sasakawa's visit has occasioned a 180-degree shift in the government's attitude. Now, we can head into the field without hesitation. We can see things for ourselves and analyze the situation, so what needs to get done when will become clear. We'll compile the findings of our survey work and submit a report to the Nippon Foundation. Then we can decide how to proceed with concrete measures for eradicating the disease."

"We hear that Malawi has leprosy colonies besides Utale."

"It has five other colonies. All of them are under the management of nonprofit organizations. [The health ministry officials] told us that Catholic missionaries are running the facility that they showed us in Utale as a leprosy colony. In fact, it's just an ordinary hospital."

"What?"

"It's just a hospital."

I was speechless. The government had created a Potemkin village in Utale. It had assembled all those patients and former patients from actual leprosy colonies just for our visit. That the government had elected to deceive the WHO ambassador was beyond belief. And we had swallowed the whole story, hook, line, and sinker. Yet our visit had yielded results nonetheless. I had a feeling like we'd acted out some kind of parable.

4

A DANCING AMBASSADOR IN A PYGMY JUNGLE
CENTRAL AFRICAN REPUBLIC

Our party headed from Malawi to the Central African Republic, traveling back through Ethiopia. We deplaned at 8 p.m. in Addis Ababa Bole International Airport's alpine-thin atmosphere and spent the night at the city's Hilton. Our flight left at nine o'clock in Addis Ababa's bracing morning air and took us to the Central African Republic capital of Bangui. That city, the Central African Republic's largest, lies just north of the equator at the southern end of the nation.

"Let's switch seats," proposed Yohei. "You need to get a good look at the scenery."

I complied, sliding into Yohei's window seat. The scenery would need to wait, however, since the plane had just climbed through an opacity of cloud cover and leveled off above at cruising altitude. Yohei launched into a commentary on our destination.

"They call the terrain that stretches from the Democratic Republic of the Congo, right on the equator, to the Central African Republic 'the lungs of Africa.' It's a vast swath of rainforest that generates a massive output of oxygen and gets an immense amount of precipitation. We were in Malawi for winter there, but we'll hit midsummer where we're headed—the rainy season, to boot. The Central African Republic is little known to people around the world. This is my first visit, but I know that the place has a lot of problems."

Yohei suspended his commentary briefly to request a coffee of a cabin attendant who came to take his order.

"The nation borders Chad on the north; Sudan [now Sudan and South Sudan] on the east; the Democratic Republic of the Congo and the Republic of the Congo (Congo-Brazzaville) on the south; and Cameroon on the west. You have a basically uninterrupted swath of tropical rain forest across the

Central African Republic and the [six] nations on its periphery. That's where we encounter one problem: desertification. Desert is encroaching on the rainforest at an alarming pace—several meters a year.

"Another problem is political instability. Central African Republic governments have succumbed repeatedly to coups d'état and civil war since the country won independence from France in 1960. The current president, François Bozizé [deposed in March 2013], seized power with the assistance of the Chadian government while his predecessor was out of the country. He's been president for eight years, but he's had to contend almost continuously with military action by antigovernment forces, so I haven't had the chance until now to visit the nation."

I expressed befuddlement at the notion of such a nation having attained the WHO's "elimination" benchmark for leprosy: less than 1 active case per 10,000 population.

"They reached the benchmark on a nationwide basis in 2005," confirmed Yohei. "But they're still short of the target in 4 of their 16 prefectures. The WHO reports that they had 235 new cases in 2010 and that they had 0.52 active cases per 10,000 population. Political instability takes a toll, of course, on the priority allocated to health administration, and reports from the field suggest that the number of cases is trending upward somewhat.

A dancing welcome

Lush verdure filled my window as the plane descended and broke through the clouds in our approach to Bangui M'Poko International Airport. Directly below, the Ubangi River flowed leisurely toward Bangui and on to its rendezvous, further south, with the Congo River. My heart raced at the thought of our impending encounter with pygmies.

We deplaned at two o'clock. The intense sunshine, the sweltering heat, and the drenching humidity were more than enough to remind us of our proximity to the equator. An impressive contingent turned out at the airport to welcome Yohei. Heading the contingent were three state ministers: Jean-Michel Mandaba, public health and AIDS prevention; Marguérite Pétro-Koni-Zezé, social affairs, national solidarity and gender promotion; and Gisèle Annie Nam, primary and secondary education and literacy. Joining them was the WHO's country representative, Dr. Zakaria Maiga. Dr. Landry Bide, the regional adviser at the WHO's Republic of the Congo–based regional office for Africa, had accompanied us on the plane and was also present. A delegation of journalists trained a battery of video cameras and still cameras on the arrival. Watching over things carefully were the members of a security detail, dressed in camouflage fatigues and shouldering light machine guns.

Yohei chatted briefly with the government ministers in the VIP lounge adjacent to the two-story airport building.

"We've been having heavy rains daily," smiled Mandaba. "But the skies cleared for your arrival."

"Well, I thank you for arranging the lovely weather," replied Yohei in the same jesting tone. "I'd have you know, however, that I usually bring rain."

This rejoinder elicited the intended laughter from all. Yohei had taken a liking to Mandaba, who was only 41 and had demonstrated a commitment to his work at the health ministry.

"We know that you are tired from the long journey, but could you please spare a few words for the media representatives here today?" Mandaba requested. Yohei gladly delivered his usual spiel: leprosy is a curable disease, it's no different from tuberculosis or malaria or any other infectious disease, those who have contracted leprosy can receive medicine free of charge from the government, any discrimination against persons affected by leprosy is the product of misunderstanding.

I lingered in the lounge after Yohei stepped out, but I dashed out at the sound of him calling me excitedly. A clamor of drumming and singing had arisen beside the airport. About 20 men and women dressed in colorful ethnic garb were singing while doing a stomp dance. "Dressed," to be sure, overstates the case somewhat, since the men concealed only their loins and the women only their loins and breasts.

"This is a dance of welcome," explained Mandaba. The music was apparently improvisational, since the words "Sasakawa, Sasakawa" were audible among the lyrics. Each performer took their turn dancing to the forefront and enunciating those lyrics while stomping the ground. Here, to the accompaniment of djembe percussion, was an evocation of the energy of the earth. The vitality of the performance imparted welcome vigor to our travel-weary bodies.

So invigorated was Yohei's body that he grabbed the hands of a male dancer and joined in the stomp dancing. The rest of us in his party clapped hands in time with the music.

"I've never had a welcome like this before," exuded a sweaty Yohei after his dancing.

Yohei would soon enjoy an encounter more gratifying still.

"Oh, look who's here," he observed happily.

Waiting on the far side of the performers to meet with Yohei were about 20 leprosy patients and former patients. They were men and women of a broad range in age. Their struggle with the disease was readily apparent. Standing in a row, the patients and former patients had the collective appearance of a sagging fence. Several stood at awkward angles, favoring one leg or the other. Some were using crutches. Two males propped up a woman—perhaps their mother, possibly their grandmother—who had apparently lost the use of her legs. On the ground before her was a crude wooden push cart that she presumably used for mobility.

"They've turned out for this day!" gushed Yohei in gratitude.

He greeted each in turn, shaking hands and delivering robust hugs. Then, he addressed the entire group.

"Thank you for turning out like this today. I've been looking forward to this opportunity to meet you. Your government representatives and I will discuss ways to improve your lot, and we'll do everything possible to make that happen."

Yohei next went back to the elderly woman and grasped her deformed hands.

"Getting around with those legs can't be easy. Thank you for coming today."

The gathering was clearly something that the government had organized. But we took that as a positive sign. Someone in the government, we surmised, was acting on a newfound commitment to eliminating prejudice and discrimination.

We got into cars for the ride to our lodging and the welcome chance to change out of our travel wear. Leading our column was a BMW motorcycle driven by a soldier who stood more than two meters tall. Immediately behind him and bringing up the rear were military trucks that carried in their beds troops armed with light machine guns.

The road into the city from the airport was an unpaved strip of red earth that carried us through dark-green forest. We passed a bustling marketplace and then caught sight of a village beyond the trees. A hill came into view behind the village. A broad road zigzagged up a slope that had been cut in the hillside. It ended at a large white structure that stood midway up the hill: the National Assembly building.

A narrow unpaved path continued up the hill behind the modern-looking home of the legislature through terraced fields. A lone farmer was visible walking down the path at a leisurely pace. Our lodging, the National Guest House, faced the hill on which the National Assembly building perched. From the outside, it had the forbidding look of a prison. Surrounding the complex was a thick concrete wall fully five meters tall. We looked in vain for a gate.

The only way in, we discovered, was a squeeze-through orifice that admitted just one person at a time.

Inside the wall were several single-story cottages of whitewashed wood and concrete and, in the center, a dining hall tended by two young women. My room, which stood across from Yohei's, was a little more than 10 square meters and offered a narrow single bed and a small desk. A small window high on the wall was the only source of natural light. Eager for a respite from the oppressive heat, I pushed the switch to turn on the air conditioner, but nothing happened. I sought relief in the shower, but the feeble water pressure produced barely a trickle. Slumber in this cell, I could see, would be a sweaty ordeal.

A continental challenge

We followed the giant on the BMW to the WHO's country office at 4:30 in the afternoon. Vehicles loaded with armed soldiers again joined our column to provide protection. The WHO office occupied a white, two-story building of European architecture that stood amid shady trees. Our hosts led us into a comfortable, air-conditioned work space where we received an orientation from Dr. Maiga. He reported that no incidents had occurred in Bangui "since June 20" but refrained ominously from touching on whatever had occurred on or up to that date. Maiga reassured us that Bangui ranked level 2 in the UN Security Level System, where level 1 indicates the least dangerous environment and level 6 the most dangerous.

"The government of the Central African Republic will ensure your safety while you are here," continued Maiga. "And I pray that you will have a safe stay. But things can happen here, and I'll provide you with contact information for me and for my colleague." Maiga motioned toward the man seated next to him and added, "He is in charge of our leprosy-control efforts."

We then moved to a meeting room, where 10 journalists sat on the window side of a long table and seven WHO staffers sat along the other side. Maiga introduced the members of his team, starting with his personal assistant. Five of the WHO staffers were female: Maiga's personal assistant, an administrator, and three physicians. One of the female physicians was responsible for efforts to eradicate AIDS, another for measures to promote health management in households, and the third for work to distribute pharmaceuticals. The two male staffers were a physician responsible for work in fighting neglected tropical diseases—the man Maiga had introduced earlier—and the office accountant.

Yohei and the rest of us from Japan then introduced ourselves. Dr. Bide followed with a well-prepared, passionate, and personal summary of the battle against leprosy in the region.

"Dr. Maiga has been a role model for me in my work," said Bide. "As for Yohei Sasakawa, he is a highly influential person in Japan, and he is here today as the WHO goodwill ambassador for the elimination of leprosy.

"Ambassador Sasakawa is a torchbearer for us at the WHO. He has stridden in the vanguard of our battle against leprosy here in Africa and in nations around the world. Now, the ambassador is tackling a new challenge. That challenge is one of moving beyond bringing leprosy under control to eradicating it completely. Ambassador Sasakawa is a great man, but his commitment to his quest is simple and straightforward. Please take this opportunity to share with him frankly the issues that you face in your work in the Central African Republic."

The physician responsible for leprosy-control efforts reiterated the summary that I had heard on the plane from Yohei: the Central African Republic had attained the WHO's elimination benchmark of less than 1 active case per 10,000 population on a nationwide basis, but the prevalence of the disease exceeded the benchmark in 4 of the nation's 16 prefectures. He showed us a map on which those prefectures appeared in red. They were Ombella-M'Poko, where we were assembled in Bangui; two prefectures to the northeast; and Lobaye, which lies on the southwest side of Ombella-M'Poko and borders the Republic of the Congo to the south. Our itinerary called for a visit the next day to a pygmy community in Lobaye.

"Pygmies have a high prevalence of leprosy," continued the physician. "Higher than 1 per 10,000 population. To put it precisely, the prevalence is 1.84 per 10,000."

"The WHO conducted a survey across Africa in 2000," interjected Bide, "and it revealed that leprosy was still not under control in 12 nations on the continent. But a follow-up survey five years later found that all of those nations had brought the disease under control. Twenty years of hard work in African nations had shrunk the rolls of active cases by 1.5 million. However, the rate of prevalence has edged upward slightly in recent years in a few African nations, including the Central African Republic."

Bide reported that the WHO had confirmed an uptick in the rate of leprosy incidence in 2008, that it had detected evidence subsequently of a further upturn, and that those findings had prompted the WHO to undertake a new survey. On that note, he lauded the timing of Yohei's visit.

"Ambassador Sasakawa has finally made his way to this nation that the world has abandoned, and this visit is not by any means too late. Please allow me to provide some perspective.

"This is not the only nation where leprosy's prevalence is rising. In the south of Africa, Botswana was getting only 1 or 2 new cases a year, but the health authorities there reported 43 new cases last year. Leprosy is gaining momentum all across the continent, and contracting the disease remains a severely traumatic experience for the persons affected. Left untreated, leprosy causes disfigurement and invites discrimination. That's an especially lamentable facet of leprosy: outward traces can remain and occasion discrimination even after the disease has been cured."

Yohei's turn came to talk, and he began with a hearty expression of gratitude.

"Let me begin by thanking all of you who took part in bringing about this visit to your nation. You have overcome daunting obstacles in working to improve the health of your fellow citizens. And you have my deepest gratitude and my great admiration.

"I have traveled the world in my fight against leprosy. My experience has reaffirmed for me a simple truth: all people born into this world, wherever they reside, have the right to live as equals. A person might contract a serious disease. But that person has the right to live. And if we have a cure for that person's disease, can we be forgiven for failing to act. Everyone has the right to health and peace of mind.

"My work has included dealing with nearly all of the principal agencies at the United Nations. And I can assure you that the one that interacts most closely with people in each nation is the World Health Organization. My mission as the WHO ambassador is to help eliminate leprosy from the African continent and from the earth and to help shape a social environment that is open and receptive to former leprosy patients."

What I witnessed in that meeting room was a revelation. Most of the people in the room were seeing and hearing Yohei for the first time. Gazing into their intent faces, I grasped anew the influence that he wielded as the WHO goodwill ambassador. He had traveled halfway around the world to see a nation where leprosy was ostensibly under control. Merely "under control" was wholly unsatisfactory for Yohei where the rate of incidence was rising, however modest the upturn.

These people had concerns more pressing than leprosy. They were initially skeptical about Yohei's passion for fighting leprosy and, truth be told, the value of the day's meeting. They knew, of course, that annual disbursals from his Nippon Foundation were funding the WHO's leprosy-control program. They knew, too, that those disbursals were covering the cost of distributing the multidrug therapy kits and were paying the salaries of numerous health officers at WHO facilities around the world. And they surely knew that Yohei had no pecuniary interest in the quest against leprosy. They were more concerned, however, with fending off the Ebola hemorrhagic fever viruses that lurked in their rainforest and with stopping the spread of HIV and AIDS.

Yohei's presentation went right to the heart of his listeners' doubts.

"I know that you have your doubts about our cause. You wonder why you would take time in your daily work to tackle leprosy, which is less prevalent than malaria. The reason is that leprosy is a disease that presents special challenges. With other diseases, persons who contract the diseases take the initiative in seeking treatment. But with leprosy, medical care providers need to seek out the persons afflicted with the disease. That's because leprosy has occasioned discrimination since before the days of the Old Testament. It's because society treats the afflicted persons as diseased individuals even after they have been cured and bars them from reentering the community. It's because we still have numerous people who regard leprosy as divine punishment.

"Changing attitudes toward leprosy will hinge on our success in instilling in national leaders a commitment to eradicating the disease. In the Central African Republic, you at the WHO need to develop a good working relationship with the health ministry for tackling leprosy. I have come in the spirit of helping to build that relationship."

Yohei then turned to the journalists. He urged them to help raise awareness of the importance of public sanitation. Yohei invited them to cover his activity during his stay in the Central African Republic. And he called on them to propagate an accurate understanding of leprosy among everyone in the Central African Republic. Yohei reiterated that leprosy is curable and that medicine for treating the disease is available free of charge. He concluded with a plea for disseminating the message that discriminating against persons affected by leprosy is evil.

"We have a serious problem," chimed in Maiga forcefully, "if a disease is out there and people are hiding its existence."

The journalists rose to leave, and Yohei shook hands with each as they made their way out. Outside, the noise of the insects had crescendoed into a clamor. The clock showed six o'clock.

I applied insect repellent from head to toe before going to bed, and the sticky coating combined with surging perspiration to prevent me from enjoying much in the way of slumber. Yohei looked every bit the happy camper, though, as he appeared in the dining room the next morning. Our travel instructions for the Central African Republic included firm instructions not to eat raw vegetables. No cooked vegetables appeared, however, on the table. The menu consisted only of dry bread, cassava, and desiccated roast chicken.

Fortified by what had passed for breakfast, we left the hotel at 7:30 and met with Mandaba at the health ministry to convey Yohei's concerns and to reconfirm our schedule. Yohei asked the minister to address the overall increase in incidence and to step up control measures in the four prefectures that had not attained the WHO's elimination benchmark. And he repeated his call for efforts to eliminate discrimination against persons affected by leprosy.

Yohei reminded Mandaba that Bide, who was present, was the officer responsible for leprosy at the WHO's regional office for Africa. He told the minister that Bide had been a valuable adviser to him in the struggle against leprosy. Yohei urged Mandaba to consult with Bide in working to eliminate leprosy in the Central African Republic. He continued talking through a power outage that occurred during the discussion.

Mandaba pledged to follow Yohei's instructions in tackling leprosy in the four prefectures where its prevalence remained above the WHO's benchmark and to look to Bide for leadership in bringing the disease under control there. He informed us, evincing happy surprise, that Yohei's remarks at the airport the previous day had received prominent television coverage.

"Everyone, including government figures, follows the TV news coverage," Mandaba assured Yohei. "Your remarks also received radio and newspaper coverage. They were a powerful wake-up call for our nation. Your message resounded with government figures and with ordinary citizens. 'Leprosy is just another disease, like tuberculosis or malaria. We mustn't discriminate against the patients or former patients.'"

A palace in the forest depths

Mandaba accompanied Yohei and the rest of us on our sojourn into the jungle to visit a village. It would be his first interchange with the pygmies there. We got into the four Land Cruisers provided by the WHO and by the health ministry and departed from the ministry at nine o'clock. As before, the giant on the BMW led the way, and trucks loaded with armed soldiers accompanied us to provide security.

Our caravan was out of Bangui in the blink of an eye. No power poles stood along the road. Not a single line stretched overhead.

"The villages around here don't have electricity, gas, or water," said our driver.

Children pushed makeshift carts heaped with dry branches along the side of the road. Adults conveyed logs on similar contraptions. We learned from the driver that the wood was for fuel.

"They're taking it to sell in Bangui," continued the driver. "Parts of Bangui are also without electricity or gas."

I mentioned that I was curious about the sunny weather we'd had since our arrival the previous day. After all, this was supposed to be the rainy season. The driver assured me that they'd had an especially heavy rain on the day before our arrival. He then provided some information about the pygmies that we were about to encounter.

"The pygmies don't come out of the forest during the rainy season. They eat the caterpillars that fall out of the tree branches. They yank the caterpillars in half and dig out the insides. They just eat the outside. They get protein that way."

"Do they eat the caterpillars raw?" I asked.

"No, no. They cook everything first in hot water or oil. Bananas are the main food for the village five or six kilometers ahead. The bananas are small, and they're too bitter to eat raw, so the pygmies fry them first."

Our unpaved road over the red earth was bumpy, and the handwriting of my notes was so jumpy that I wondered if I'd be able to read it later. The trees of the forest attained massive dimensions and shut out the sunlight on both sides of the road.

"Ugandan poachers come from the east to hunt our elephants. They come for the ivory."

Just as the driver had spit out this non sequitur for our edification, a Chinese-language billboard popped into view.

"What's that?! It's Chinese, right?" I asked the driver.

"Chinese are teaching people around here how to grow rice. They're looking for land to buy, the Chinese are."

The driver didn't sound very happy about the Chinese. Another site changed the subject, however, a little further up the road.

"What in the world...?!"

I was at a loss for words. Standing in a sudden clearing in the otherwise dense forest was an imposing, palace-like structure of stunning scale. The baroque architecture was utterly out of place in this remote corner of a prodigiously impoverished nation.

"It's the ruins of Berengo Palace," explained the driver. "President [Jean-Bédel] Bokassa proclaimed himself Emperor Bokassa I and built this palace.

We're in an area called Berengo. Nearby is the village of Bobangui, where Bokassa was born.

Bokassa had served with distinction in the French military in Africa, Europe, and Indochina. He consolidated power in the Central African Republic, which won independence from France in 1960, as the head of the nation's military. That was under the first president, who was a distant cousin. Bokassa deposed his cousin in a coup d'état in 1966 and became the second president. He named himself president for life in 1972 and, as the driver said, emperor in 1976.

The coronation ceremony that Bokassa staged in Bangui in 1977 cost a reported $25 million, equivalent to the nation's annual budget. Bokassa became infamous for the decadence epitomized by the coronation and, even more, for cruelty that was extreme even by the standards of African dictators. Especially appalling was the Bokassa-supervised slaughter of children who protested against a government mandate that they buy expensive school uniforms. That proved too much for the French government, which had formerly supported the dictator and which subsequently sponsored a coup that restored his predecessor to power.

"We have no shoes"

Our caravan passed by a large lumber mill a little after 10 o'clock. The ambient luminosity mounted in the openness that had been created by clear-cutting, though burning in advance of cultivation had charred the landscape black. People appeared on the scene, and they were small. Across from the charred, clear-cut aftermath was a meadow where what appeared to be cones of cut grass stood drying in the sun. But what we took initially for haystacks turned out to be dwellings—grass huts.

Some of the people crouched around fires, cooking. Some were standing, but even erect, they were of childlike stature. We had arrived at the Lobaye Prefecture village of Kaka. A crowd gathered in the clearing on the left side of the road. Everyone was wearing T-shirts. Some members of the crowd were pygmies, the tallest of whom stood no higher than my navel. Some, including the village headman, were of normal stature.

The headman stepped forward to greet Yohei and his party. He urged us toward a bamboo awning that the villagers had apparently erected for our visit. About 40 pygmies were standing under the awning. Sitting and standing apart from them in the shade of trees were two groups of pygmies instantly recognizable as victims of leprosy. We walked over to and through those two groups.

One person was missing a leg, another an arm. Yet another was missing a foot and leaned, visibly in pain, on crutches and a single bare foot. These and others in the community who had contracted leprosy had not known that medicine was available to treat their affliction, had not known to seek medical care, had not known that they had a disease called leprosy. Yohei shook hands with each in turn and then, at the urging of our hosts, took a seat at an elevated spot under the awning. He had changed into local ethnic garb.

We then heard the sound of shouting, followed by an explosion of bells and percussion. Several of the younger members of the crowd proceeded into the clearing and started performing a dance of welcome. The dancers joined hands in two, then three concentric rings and sang something like "Ay, ay, ay." They moved in and out as they danced, causing their concentric circles to undulate in some sort of primeval pattern. Children joined in, dilating the rings. Birds in the vicinity, as if awakened by the ruckus, began singing, too. The avian voices were strident, louder even than the people's in the remarkable admixture of timbres.

Our pulses were still racing as the performance segued into greetings by the village headman, by the mayor of a nearby city, and by a physician responsible for the district.

We talked with a member of a group of Belgian nuns who were working as nurses in the village. "We've been working in the Central Africa Republic since 1985 and happened onto this village about a year ago. The conditions here were so appalling that we decided to move here and do what we could."

The headman and mayor informed us lots of people in their village and city had AIDS or HIV. They appealed to Mandaba and to Bide for assistance in coping with those life-threatening scourges, too. A nun joined in the appeal, speaking passionately.

"Sasakawa-san and you here from the WHO and from the health ministry, please lend an ear to the voices of the patients here."

Someone passed the microphone to a pygmy who had been among the dancers and was now sitting under the awning. He could barely grasp it, though, on account of his disfigured hands.

"Sasakawa-san," the man began, "thank you for coming. We who have leprosy are at an extremely painful stage. We didn't know about the disease, but it has deformed our bodies like this. We are grateful to you for your concern and for your visit. We hope that we will get over this disease. We want the people in the government to know that we want to get well. We want to recover and get on with our lives. But we have no shoes. Please give us shoes."

The speaker's feet were white, devoid of pigment. His left foot was especially lacking in life, and I suspected that it was numb. Another man had risen but was standing with difficulty. A tiny woman whom I supposed to be his wife stood by his side. She spoke on his behalf.

"Coming down with this disease was a huge shock. We are extremely sad. It attacked our fingers and our feet first. Then, we got worse and worse. Now, we can't even hold a nut. Our legs are bad, too. We have one request. Please give us shoes."

The fingers on her hands and on the man's hands were frozen at awkward angles. Their legs had deteriorated to the point of requiring amputation. The nuns had discovered them living in the forest. Neither the man nor the woman had realized that their worsening condition was due to disease. The thought of seeking medical assistance had never entered their minds. Even if it had, no medical facilities were to be found in or anywhere near their forest abode. They finally learned the truth of their disease from the nuns, when it had progressed too far to avoid serious aftereffects.

Lobaye has a population of about 280,000, and it had 52 active cases of leprosy on its official rolls at the time of our visit. That meant 1.84 per 10,000 population, which exceeded the WHO's elimination benchmark of 1 per 10,000 population. And anyone could see that the actual incidence was surely higher still. The nuns were the only source of findings about leprosy among the pygmies of this community, and they were hardly in a position to gather comprehensive survey data.

The pygmies, who were of a group known as the Aka, relied on their feet to get around in the forest. They all went barefoot, which meant walking painfully on leprosy-caused sores on the soles of their feet.

Mandaba took the microphone to address the gathering, and the youthful minister's countenance revealed an epiphany.

"Leprosy sufferers, Chairman Sasakawa, WHO representatives, what I have heard here from persons afflicted by leprosy has been an awakening. Seeing the Nippon Foundation chairman here has reminded me that we need to do more to eradicate leprosy in our nation. This has also been an opportunity to recognize anew the importance of eliminating discrimination. Chairman Sasakawa took the hand of each leprosy sufferer. I take that as a message that we mustn't discriminate against such individuals.

"The chairman also imparted another important message. In taking the hand of each person, he dispelled our fear of the disease. Chairman Sasakawa came all the way to our nation to hear firsthand the cries for help of leprosy sufferers here. We from the government have also heard those cries. Representatives of the prefectural government of Lobaye, thank you for organizing this gathering. Let us go forward from this day and foster understanding of leprosy among the people of our nation."

An impressive honesty was audible in the young minister's remarks. Mandaba acknowledged the "fear of the disease" and of its awful symptoms, which invite notions of evil spells. His readiness to address openly the widespread revulsion toward leprosy was refreshing and promising. Mandaba confessed that he had formerly been unwilling to do as Yohei had in taking the hands of leprosy sufferers. But Yohei had dispersed that resistance, the minister said, through his example. Mandaba went on to call for eliminating discrimination. His heartfelt remarks earned vigorous applause from Yohei, who then bowed to the headman and to the mayor and addressed the gathering.

"Villagers, I am delighted at this opportunity to see you today, especially those of you who have struggled with leprosy. You might not know anything about my nation, Japan, but it is the same as your nation. When the sun sets, the moon rises. I live under that moon, the same moon that you see in your sky. This is what I think: the world is one big house, and all people are brothers and sisters, including healthy people and people with health problems. Today, I am extremely happy to have met more of my brothers and sisters."

Yohei stepped out from under the awning and into the sun, where his face was readily visible to all.

"I have exchanged handshakes and hugs with persons around the world," he continued, "who have the same disease that you have. And look, I have not contracted the disease. Leprosy is simply not very contagious. It is just a disease like any other. People need to learn that prejudice and discrimination against individuals who have leprosy is wrong. I had the good fortune to meet with you today and to talk with some of you who have serious aftereffects of the disease. I have been sad to learn that the treatment for curing the disease is not widely available here.

"As you can see, the minister for public health and AIDS prevention is with us today. Please see that today marks the beginning of a stepped-up battle against leprosy. That battle will begin with measures to put in place sanitary conditions for providing care to ameliorate your pain and to make you as comfortable as possible."

Yohei paused here for effect.

"On that note, let me tell you that I was amazed at how wonderfully you dance. I will stop talking now, and I hope that you will teach me your dance steps."

The pygmies smiled and applauded. Yohei then concluded with a call to action: "All right, let's dance!"

This triggered another explosion of bells and percussion. The young pygmies gathered again in concentric circles in the clearing, and Yohei jumped into the middle. Among the dancers were several who had leprosy or had recovered from the disease. Yohei joined hands with some of them and executed a series of jumps. Mandaba also got into the act, dancing hand in hand with leprosy victims. I caught a glimpse of his face as he looked toward Yohei, and he was grinning from ear to ear.

Reflections on the encounter with the pygmies

The nuns showed us a clinic that the Catholic Church ran in a building nearby. They explained that it had facilities to accommodate inpatient care but that no one was staying there as an inpatient. A physician stationed in the vicinity by the health ministry would comb the forest regularly in search of leprosy victims, but the pygmies would flee in advance of his arrival. If word got out that someone was bringing food, the pygmies might well gather to partake of the treat, the nuns speculated. But news of a physician looking for sick people had the opposite effect.

No one stayed at the clinic, the nuns explained, because it didn't provide meals. Yohei's visit had drawn a turnout because the village headman and the nuns had announced that they would serve meals to all comers. That announcement proved persuasive, and pygmies had begun gathering on the previous day for the event.

"The pygmies ordinarily dance stark naked," Yohei confided to me as he wiped the sweat off his face after his turn on the "dance floor." "But they received instructions to put on clothes on our account."

"Maybe you should have taken off your clothes," I kidded.

"You're absolutely right. I'm ready, whatever it takes."

"Where do you go from here?"

"The foundation will work directly with these nuns. Giving them ¥1 million will work wonders here. If we tried to send the money through the government, it would all end up in the hands of the wrong people."

Yohei apparently mistrusted even the young health minister, who appeared so sincere. And that was only natural. The president at the time had seized power from his predecessor through a military uprising and had suppressed opposition through continued military action. Anyone in power was unlikely to be indifferent to the wealth that accrued from the nation's diamonds, uranium, and other mineral resources. How long they would be in power was yet another issue. Sporadic unrest persisted across the countryside, and another coup d'état could be just a matter of time. In short, I could easily understand why Yohei was inclined to work directly with the nuns.

As the gathering was dispersing, Yohei wandered onto a grassy area across from the clearing and the road. The pygmies had erected several simple huts of brush there. A family of five was clustered around a fire in one of the huts, cooking cassava in a metal pot. Another family was eating leftovers from the meal provided by the headman and nuns and was eating them out of a pot. One pygmy was chomping on a chicken neck.

Yohei discovered among the pygmies an albino boy. Stark naked, he had not taken part in the festivities and was waiting for whatever morsels the others saw fit to leave for him to eat. The sight called into question my assumptions about the egalitarian stance that I had associated with pygmy society. Albinism incurred persecution all across sub-Saharan Africa. People sometimes even killed and dismembered albinos in the belief that the limbs and other body parts imparted magical powers.

Aka society was, like any society, a complex network of interactions, including discriminatory relationships. It nonetheless furnished ample food for thought about peoples' interaction with the natural environment. The Aka pygmies that had gathered for Yohei's visit would soon slip back into the forest and resume their premodern mode of living. To be sure, they lacked access to the comforts of our monetary economy, including medicine. They enjoyed a freedom, however, that we abandoned long ago in exchange for the presumed benefits of industrialization.

The Aka exhibited none of the prejudice against leprosy that blighted other societies. I understood that to reflect a worldview that accepted disease as part of the natural cycle of life. The Aka, their treatment of albinism notwithstanding, had largely avoided the social stratification that accompanies modernization and, especially, industrialization. They were as one with nature as I could imagine any group of humans could be. Each of them was as a leaf on a tree of their forest home, each as a droplet of moisture that flowed through the cycle of life.

> *Simply listening*
> *Would I abandon myself*
> *To the here and now*
>
> *One with the raindrops would I*
> *Trickle downward from the eaves*

Seeing how the pygmies lived as one with nature brought to mind this poem by the Japanese zen monk Eihei Dogen (1200–1253). Embracing the culture of scientific rationalism has been a Faustian bargain for us in Western society, including Japan. In return for the creature comforts imparted by modern technology, we have countenanced separation from the natural world.

Sharing time and place with the pygmies, who retained their connection with that world, occasioned an atavistic rediscovery of unity with nature. Accompanying that rediscovery, however, was a melancholy realization: We could provide the pygmies with some of the attainments of Western culture, but the benefits would be only temporary unless the recipients saw fit to take up residence in our world. The offer of meals might attract pygmies to the clinic, but that very offer could cause frictions as the pygmies struggled to abide by their tradition of sharing equally. Our good intentions would then be disrupting, rather than enhancing, their lives.

This was Yohei's second encounter with pygmies. He had visited a jungle pygmy village in the Democratic Republic of the Congo three and a half years earlier, in November 2007. That encounter had sowed doubt in his mind similar to what I was experiencing in the Central African Republic. Yohei realized in the Congo that his ostensible altruism implied an assumption of cultural superiority. He realized, too, that imposing his values on the pygmies could have the effect of destroying their culture. Those realizations carried him further in his cultural awakening. He reflected on that awakening in the car on the way back to Bangui.

"The pygmies in the [Democratic Republic of the] Congo long suffered discrimination and oppression under the Bantu people, who are of standard height. For example, the Bantu used them as forced labor in agriculture. The Catholic Church tried to help, building schools for the pygmies. A priest boasted to me that 5,000 pygmy children had attended the schools and that 5 of them had gone on to become teachers. To tell you the truth, I've got mixed feelings about what he was describing.

"Pygmies coexist harmoniously with the forest ecology. They take only what they need to subsist and then move on. Their nomadic lifestyle is a model of environmental sustainability. I question whether steering them into a stationary lifestyle and providing them with education is really consistent with the natural order. My suspicion is that they would soon succumb to the capitalism and monetary economics of the West and to a greedy materialism."

The issues that were troubling Yohei are bigger, of course, than the problems of the pygmies. Yohei has traveled repeatedly, for instance, to

Rohingya Islamic communities in Myanmar that have suffered persecution from the Buddhist majority.

"They might be poor, but they retain a fierce pride," marveled Yohei, "in their culture. That's a big takeaway for me from every visit. We need to be careful not to wound their pride in the way we distribute the pharmaceutical bounty of our industrial civilization. Any hint of condescension is out of the question.

"Here, the pygmies pulled out all the stops in displaying hospitality, and I made a point of accepting that hospitality in full. I remain as committed as ever to curing disease and to preventing disease. But I'm also serious about the need to avoid damaging the pygmies' symbiosis with the forest ecology. I really don't know how we ought to proceed here."

Our convoy was nearing the Berengo Palace. We sped past with nary another thought for the monstrosity.

Superstition as a wellspring of prejudice

Yohei and Maiga paid a visit the next morning on Prime Minister Faustin-Archange Touadéra. His office was in a building beside the National Assembly building midway up the hill that stood before our hotel. The building had no elevator, so we walked up a spiral staircase to Touadéra's office on the top floor.

Maiga asked the prime minister to step up leprosy-control work in a two-step sequence: devote priority to the prefectures where the incidence remained above the WHO's elimination benchmark and strive subsequently to reduce the rate of incidence to zero nationwide. He noted that the number of undiscovered cases appeared to be especially large among the pygmies. Maiga wanted the prime minister to understand that poor sanitation and poor nutrition are contributing factors in the incidence of leprosy and other diseases. He called for distributing soap and food to the pygmies to improve their sanitary and dietary conditions.

"Having the [pygmy] children attend school with other children is especially useful," added Maiga. "It's a good way to inculcate an understanding of the importance of good sanitary practices."

Touadéra thanked Yohei for coming to the Central African Republic. The prime minister said that he had received a report from Mandaba about the visit to the pygmy community and that he had found it moving. He pledged to work with the WHO to control leprosy in the four prefectures where its incidence remained above the benchmark. And he affirmed a commitment to continue fighting the disease until it had been eradicated completely.

Yohei was pleasantly surprised by the passion evinced by the prime minister. Touadéra went so far as to cite the need for putting in place a support framework for disabled former patients. He had clearly given thought, meanwhile, to the need for providing pygmy children with schooling. The prime minister mused about the possibility of securing funding to offset the cost of commuting to school.

"Shaping the right environment can curtail discrimination," Touadéra stated emphatically. "I look forward to working with the WHO to carry out sound policy initiatives. Please understand, however, that the four prefectures in question also have high incidences of fatal diseases, such as malaria, AIDS, and tuberculosis. We need to work to eradicate those diseases, as well as leprosy. The same individuals can overcome leprosy only to contract malaria or even AIDS. So we need a comprehensive preventative program.

"The political unrest that has rocked this nation for too long has ended. We can turn our attention now to fighting poverty. Eighty percent of our working population is engaged in agriculture. So I am eager to launch a large-scale development program for the agricultural sector. That would improve nutrition and reduce the incidence of tragic diseases, as well as lifting people out of poverty."

Yohei expressed hearty agreement with the thoughts voiced by the prime minister. He noted that 70% of the African workforce overall is engaged in agriculture and seconded Touadéra's thoughts about improvements in agricultural standards of living as essential in fighting serious diseases. Yohei introduced the Sasakawa Global 2000 project, a wide-ranging initiative for increasing food self-sufficiency in sub-Saharan Africa by raising agricultural productivity and incomes. He informed Touadéra that the project's annual convention would take place in Mali in the coming November and asked the prime minister to dispatch his agriculture minister to the gathering.

Touadéra listened intently and, shaking hands forcefully, assured his guest that the government would dispatch a suitable representative to the gathering in Mali.

Yohei's schedule for the day also included meetings with the speaker of the national assembly and with the minister for social affairs, national solidarity, and gender promotion, who had greeted him at the airport. Those meetings yielded hints of a bill for prohibiting leprosy-related discrimination and an increase in the budget for measures aimed at controlling the disease. Yohei had hoped to secure a few moments with the president, but a meeting proved impossible.

The next day, Yohei visited the ministry of education, where he met with the ministers responsible for national education, higher education, and research; for technical and vocational education and training; and for primary and secondary education and literacy. He secured agreement from the latter, who had also greeted him at the airport, to include sanitation in school curricula. The minister for technical and vocational education and training, who we learned taught at a university, had welcome news for Yohei. He reported that the Central African Republic would participate in Sasakawa Global 2000.

Yohei was painfully familiar with the struggles and frustrations that accompany the task of nation building amid chronically insufficient budgets. He offered a word of advice to the minister responsible for technical and vocational education and training, Djibrine Sall.

"We hear from the wise that we need to bring a perspective of 1 year to cultivating crops, 10 years to cultivating trees, and 100 years to cultivating people. You naturally want to see results sooner than a century down the line as you work to nurture human resources. But you need to frame your goals across a span of decades, monitor your progress annually, and make adjustments as necessary to keep your program on track.

"Nurturing human resources is especially important in working to increase output and reduce poverty in the agricultural sector. Progress toward that goal will contribute greatly toward enriching your nation. It will also contribute greatly to lowering the incidence of tragic diseases."

Sall clearly welcomed the input, and Yohei was in good spirits as we headed for his next appointment at the UN Integrated Peacebuilding Office in Bangui. His mood darkened, however, at what he heard there from Margaret Vogt, the UN special representative and head of the office. Vogt was well aware of the UN declaration that called for ending discrimination against persons affected by leprosy, and she applauded Yohei's efforts to raise government and media awareness of that issue in the Central African Republic. She was equally aware, however, of a problem unique to that nation and to several other sub-Saharan nations, which she described to Yohei.

"Pervasive superstitions are an obstacle to propagating human rights here and throughout the primitive societies of sub-Saharan Africa. Those superstitions can include regarding disabled persons, sickly women, and victims of leprosy as receptacles of evil spirits. That can entail all manner of abuse, even to the point of taking life. This is a truly pressing issue."

Vogt's eyes teared up as she described an issue that obviously weighed heavily on her heart. Yohei was familiar with the role of superstition in discrimination against persons affected by leprosy. He knew that superstition in the bush was a corollary to the ignorance and insensitivity exhibited by national leaders. Witness the following remark by Yoweri Museveni, the president of Uganda, in a meeting there with Yohei in 2001.

"We have no leprosy in Uganda. We discarded it in Lake Victoria."

Even discounting the feeble and inapt attempt at humor, we perceive in Museveni's remark a failure to take the problem seriously. Yohei knew from experience that most national leaders, if presented with accurate, eye-opening information, would do the right thing. He had seen that even the poorest nations could bring leprosy under control when their leaders exerted informed commitment. And he had learned that personal encounters with leaders could be opportunities for correcting misperceptions. Here are excerpts from Yohei's conversations with two other presidents.

"We in Tanzania say about bad things, 'Avoid it like leprosy.' I've used that expression a lot. But I won't use it anymore." Benjamin Mkapa, Tanzania, 2005.

"Before your visit, I was terrified of leprosy. I'd close the windows of my car when passing near a leprosarium and ask the driver to speed up. But I'll watch on television to see if you really hug the leprosy patients when you visit the leprosarium tomorrow. And if you do, I'll pay a visit on the patients, too." Rupiaha Banda, Zambia, 2009.

"You cannot imagine," Vogt assured Yohei, "how inspiring your visit has been. The media have devoted extensive coverage to the way you held the hands of the leprosy sufferers and took part in the dancing. Those images are invaluable in eliminating discrimination. No one here had ever seen anything like that before. You have shown us how things ought to be and can be."

Vogt thus accompanied her cautionary admonition about superstition with an encouraging word about the positive results of Yohei's crusade. Yohei's spirits took another hit, however, from the scene at the next stop on our itinerary.

We traveled to a health care center about 25 kilometers from Bangui that serves as one of five leprosy clinics in the Central African Republic. The center, we learned, served eight outpatients who were receiving treatment for leprosy. We were appalled to see, however, that it had no multidrug therapy (MDT) blister packs in stock and that the patient records were not up to date. The staff members present when we visited explained that the MDT blister packs were on order and that they and their colleagues had evacuated the site during recent unrest.

Yohei had set foot in 30 of the continent's 54 nations, mainly in sub-Saharan Africa. This was the first time that he had encountered an ostensible "leprosy care" facility bereft of MDT blister packs. We saw that peace and stability remained an unfulfilled dream in this nation, whatever the prime minister might say. Stable government had failed to take hold over the decades, and the victims of oppression were eager for vengeance.

The battle against leprosy had started from square one under the present government, and it would begin anew from square one under the next government. I knew better than to press Yohei further about his plans for this nation. He knew how things worked here.

5

ENTREPRENEURIAL INITIATIVE
RAIPUR (INDIA)

Our plane left Delhi's Indira Gandhi International Airport at 7:40 a.m. on September 22, 2011, and landed at Raipur Airport (now Swami Vivekananda Airport) an hour and 40 minutes later. Raipur is the capital of the east-central Indian state of Chhattisgarh. The state is 1 of 16 born in November 2000 through the partition of 10 Chhattisgarhi- and 6 Gondi-speaking districts in southeastern Madhya Pradesh. As the name suggests, Chhattisgarhi is an official language in the state, along with Hindi. The poverty rate in Chhattisgarh at the time of our visit was nearly 40%—approximately double the rate for India overall. Minority ethnic groups account for more than one-third of the population.

Yohei was making his second visit to Chhattisgarh, having visited the state previously in 2004. India had attained the WHO's "elimination" benchmark for leprosy of less than 1 active case per 10,000 population, but two states—Chhattisgarh and Bihar—remained above that level. Chhattisgarh had 4,952 active cases, which was equivalent to a prevalence rate of 1.94 cases per 10,000 population. The rate had declined greatly since Yohei's first visit, when it was 5.08.

Multiple factors accounted for Chhattisgarh's high prevalence rate of leprosy in 2004. One problem was poverty, which figures prominently in the incidence of the disease everywhere. As noted, poverty was more widespread in Chhattisgarh than in India as a whole. It is especially common among minority ethnic groups, and the large percentage of ethnic minorities in Chhattisgarh's population inflated the state's poverty rate. A lot of the members of the minority ethnic group resided, meanwhile, in remote areas where sanitation and nutrition tended to be poor and access to medical services inadequate.

Yohei recalled for me an episode that had instilled hope for progress in defeating leprosy in Chhattisgarh, the challenges notwithstanding. On his

2004 visit, he had visited a public health center in an ethnic-minority village about 30 kilometers from Raipur. Some 20 health workers had gathered there to finalize preparations for a leprosy-control campaign that would begin the next day.

The men and women gathered at the center exhibited a thorough understanding of leprosy and a good grasp of its persistence in Chhattisgarh. Their campaign would build on a well-established work regimen that included visiting patients' homes on motorcycles and bicycles. The center served a population of about 100,000. That meant that the health workers who had assembled at the health center each served an average of 5,000 people. They therefore resided at points across the state.

Yohei was impressed to hear that some of the health workers were visiting homes that were inaccessible even by bicycle. He cited a Chinese proverb by way of encouragement.

"A 100-mile journey is only half over at the 99-mile mark. We are at the halfway mark this year and next year. Let us retain our sense of urgency and carry our quest through to completion."

"We'll get the rate down to 1 person per 10,000 population by next year," pledged one of the workers confidently. The worker coupled that pledge with "a prominent Brahman in this vicinity came down with leprosy and received the multidrug therapy, which cured him completely. The only aftereffect of the disease was a minor crook in one of his little fingers, and he was extremely grateful. Leprosy strikes most broadly among impoverished people at the bottom of the social latter, but it can afflict anyone. And we provide treatment without regard for caste."

Yohei was keenly aware that Chhattisgarh remained above the WHO's elimination benchmark as he returned in 2011, and he therefore wanted to take a fresh look at conditions on the ground there. He was also aware that prejudice against persons affected by leprosy was rife in the state. That heightened his desire to encourage redoubled efforts there to bring the disease under control and to eradicate discrimination.

WHO vehicles took us the morning after our arrival for the drive to a district health center. We reached the bright, skin-colored building that housed the center in about two hours. The director of the center and lots of state health officers were on hand to greet Yohei, but the atmosphere was somehow less than ingratiating.

"How are you doing with the multidrug treatment?" Yohei asked the director. "Are you using it effectively?"

"Yes," was the terse reply.

"How many leprosy patients do you have here?"

"None."

"Really?! None? Don't you have social workers going from village to village in search of persons afflicted by the disease?"

"Even if they found someone, this center would likely be too far for the person to commute for treatment."

"Your social workers surely aren't that helpless. If they found someone with leprosy, they could bring the person here, couldn't they?"

We could see from what our hosts showed us at the health center that it had a robust inventory of multidrug therapy blister packs. The health authorities had positioned the center to provide treatment for leprosy as needed. But the passionate commitment to eliminating leprosy that Yohei had sensed in Chhattisgarh seven years earlier had cooled.

"That place serves 32,000 people," Yohei grumbled to me as we pulled away from the health center. "They're not being honest when they say they don't have any cases of leprosy. What's going on at a place like this becomes pretty clear right off. They knew that we were coming at least two days ago, and they did nothing in the way of preparations for our visit. It's a slipshod operation."

Lots of health care officers had gathered for our visit, but they were visibly uncomfortable. No one seemed to know exactly who we were or what they were supposed to do.

"The director claims that the center is too far for villagers to commute for leprosy care. But that's ridiculous. Case workers who took their jobs seriously would carry patients in as necessary. This has been a good chance to see just how lax the state government is here about leprosy control."

Yohei had a bad aftertaste in his mouth, and he wanted to get a look at more serious efforts to combat the disease. We headed back to Raipur and set out anew for the Bramba Vihar leprosy colony in the town of Bilaspur. The ride was over rough, unpaved roads and took about four hours. It would have been shorter but for the need to accommodate cows on the road. Sometimes, that meant negotiating carefully around a cow lying in our path. Sometimes, it meant stopping outright to await the passage of a bovine procession moving in the opposite direction.

The monsoon season was ostensibly ending, but the clouds had dumped heavy rain on the Bramba Vihar colony the day before our visit. Huge puddles dotted the grounds, and everything about the buildings was sopping wet. The floor in the colony's assembly hall was a swamp, but the residents nonetheless turned out en masse to welcome Yohei.

Bramba Vihar occupies land owned by the state forestry department. It dates from 1979 and had 23 households and 45 residents at the time of our visit. Bramba Vihar receives support from the Leprosy Mission, a nonprofit organization that has been fighting leprosy since 1874. The Leprosy Mission's support for the fight against leprosy spans health care, vocational training, community empowerment, legal and political advocacy, and research and training. At Bramba Vihar, the Leprosy Mission supports four groups that engage in self-reliant enterprise. The groups earn money through their enterprise and save their earnings in jointly managed bank accounts. Whatever enterprise was under way at the colony did little, however, to disguise the unmistakable aura of poverty.

Chitra Singh, the colony's leader and an affable man of middle age, welcomed Yohei and the rest of us to the community. Female residents dressed in saris of primary colors surrounded Yohei and hung floral wreaths around his neck. Singh described the struggles that the colony faced.

"We keep working on the state government, for example, to do something about this flooding in the monsoon season."

"One colony alone can only do so much," cautioned Yohei. "But if the colonies throughout Chhattisgarh join hands, you absolutely can get the state to act."

Yohei had brought along Ghasiram Bhoi, the president of the State Leprosy Rehabilitation Committee of Chhattisgarh. He took Bhoi's hand at this point and steered it into a handshake with Singh. Yohei then knelt down before a boy who was in attendance.

"Don't you have protective shoes?" Yohei asked while examining the boy's toes.

"They gave me a pair of Micro Cellular Rubber shoes," answered the youth absently.

Micro Cellular Rubber is an Indian invention. Physicians and physiotherapists at a hospital in the state of Tamil Nadu wanted to make soft, protective shoes for feet numbed by leprosy. Working with a rubber company, they developed Micro Cellular Rubber for that purpose, and shoes made from the material have been a boon to persons afflicted by leprosy and to other persons with special podiatric needs.

"So why don't you wear them? Are they difficult to walk in?"

"The rain has been horrible. Water puddles are everywhere, so I didn't wear the shoes today. I'll be able to wear them again when the rainy season is over."

Residents had set out stepping-stones to help negotiate the water puddles. The stab at landscaping was hardly sufficient, however, for the challenge at hand.

"You really ought to wear the protective shoes," chimed in a man from the Leprosy Mission. Turning to Yohei, he continued. "Only about a tenth of the residents at this colony wear shoes. The people here are in the habit of going barefoot." He then resumed his admonishment of the boy. "You've really got to wear the shoes. They protect the sores on your feet. That's what they're for."

The boy seemed to be trying to manage something in the way of rebuttal, but words failed him in a way that was painful to watch. Leprosy had deadened the nerves in his feet. That prevented him from feeling the pain that walking on his ulcered feet would ordinarily occasion. The boy therefore failed to grasp fully the concern expressed by the man from the Leprosy Mission. He epitomized the tragedy of leprosy sufferers through the ages: deadened nerves obscured damage to ulcered extremities, and infections and other problems occurred, sometimes incurring the need for amputation.

We heard from the boy that he received a stipend of 300 rupees a month— about ¥550 (around $6.50)—from the state government. He told us, too, that he commuted to a clinic for rehabilitative care, but that seemed doubtful in the light of his physical condition.

Yohei introduced Bhoi to the residents who had gathered in the assembly hall as a prominent spokesperson for former leprosy patients. He emphasized that Bhoi was a member of National Forum India (since renamed the Association of People Affected by Leprosy), as well as the president of the State Leprosy Rehabilitation Committee of Chhattisgarh. The National Forum, as described elsewhere, is an organization of some 700 leprosy colonies that advances the interests of leprosy patients and former patients. Yohei urged the residents to work with Bhoi to mobilize Chhattisgarh's colonies in pressing the state government for infrastructural improvements and other needs.

"I am not Superman," acknowledged Yohei. "But I will strive to help improve your standard of living. Those of you who suffer from severe disabilities deserve larger pensions. All of you deserve a better environment. Your young people deserve the chance to make the most of their potential in the community. I will help you tackle those goals. But we need to avoid relying on the state government for everything. We need to do what we can on our own. I was impressed to hear that you had taken the initiative in laying the stepping-stones outside. If you can array stepping- stones like that, you can also dig channels to divert the water from the rainfall."

Curiously, nearly all the residents in attendance were female. Yohei asked four girls in the front row if they were attending school. Three replied that they were. The fourth explained that she was caring for her mother. Yohei announced to the residents that he was donating $500 to the colony and asked them to decide among themselves how to use the donation.

"Half of the people here are out begging," opined Yohei grimly as we climbed into our cars to leave. "That's how it looks to me. Why else would we have seen so few men? And the girl who isn't attending school. She claimed that it was because she was caring for her mother. But you can be sure that she has another reason. I'll bet my bottom dollar that she stopped going to school after experiencing abuse from the other kids there. We see that a lot."

Yohei's demeanor suddenly brightened. He had recalled something that changed his mood for the better.

"They sent a donation after the [Great East Japan] Earthquake," Yohei related. "Persons affected by leprosy here sent a collective donation to use in the recovery effort. Seventy percent of them are beggars. We received a donation from beggars. Doesn't that blow your mind? These are people who have been thrown out of their homes and villages and who have resorted to a life of begging on city streets. Some of them are sending part of what they get from begging to their parents. We're talking about the very parents who tossed them out of their homes. Of course, they don't have the option of saving the money in bank accounts. Banks here won't open accounts for such small sums. Beggars can't get accounts. Begging is a bane on the world, and I want to eliminate it completely."

Reconstructive surgery for social rehabilitation

Dr. D. Bhatpahare, Chhattisgarh's state leprosy officer, gathered about 30 district leprosy officers to meet with Yohei while we were in Bilaspur. Chhattisgarh and Bihar were, as noted elsewhere, India's only two states where leprosy prevalence exceeded the WHO benchmark, and the prevalence rate was even higher in Chhattisgarh than in Bihar. Bhatpahare reiterated at the gathering the course of the rate in recent years.

Chhattisgarh had 11.0 confirmed cases of leprosy per 10,000 population in 2001, but determined leprosy-control efforts had reduced the prevalence rate to 1.46 in 2006. The rate had since rebounded, however, and had remained around 2. It exceeded 1 per 10,000 population in 10 of Chhattisgarh's 18 districts (now 27). Bhatpahare bemoaned the shortages of health care personnel, of teachers, of hospitals and clinics, and of equipment as reasons for leprosy's stubbornly high prevalence.

One of the district health officers noted the value of reconstructive surgery for leprosy-caused disfigurement.

"The intense discrimination that leprosy draws has, of course, a religious dimension, but the mere visibility of the aftereffects is also a big factor. I know a man whose leprosy disfigured the fingers on his left hand and who had surgery that corrected the problem. He has built a successful pottery business and is supporting a wife and three children. Letting people know about success stories like this one will call attention to the importance of proper care and lessen discrimination."

Yohei jumped at the invitation to visit the former patient, Harilal Kumhar, at his home. Earthenware pots were all about the smallish home, which doubled as a pottery workshop. Kumhar and his wife, Sarojani, and three children were the very picture of a happy family. The fingers on the potter's left hand were straight and sound.

"Scenes like this inspire hope," smiled Yohei while stroking the heads of the children.

"We are devoting high priority to reconstructive surgery for former leprosy patients," reported Bhatpahare after we left the Kumhar's home. "About 80 individuals have undergone surgery this year, and we are aiming for 100 next year. Have a look at these photos."

Bhatpahare showed Yohei "before" and "after" shots of a boy who, like the potter, had suffered disfigurement of the fingers of his left hand. In the "before" photo, the boy, on the verge of tears, is holding out the disfigured hand. In the "after" photo, the boy, smiling, is showing off his perfectly repaired hand.

"Reconstructive surgery," Bhatpahare continued, "restores smiles to people's faces. But we don't have enough personnel [to perform the surgeries]."

"We need to get the state government to act," agreed Yohei. "Mr. Bhoi and I will be calling on the state health minister today. I'll urge him to put his ministry to work on the problem."

Before we parted, Bhatpahare described encouraging progress of another kind in combating discrimination. He reported that schools in the state had supplemented their curricula with lesson material about why leprosy discrimination is wrong.

We then headed for the official residence of the state health minister, Amar Agrawal. People and cows jammed the street. This, we learned, was Agrawal's 49th birthday, and political supporters had turned out to wish the minister well. "Happy Birthday" posters were everywhere. Even the cows were getting into the act.

The minister's official residence was, in contrast with the festivities outside, a modest affair, something akin to a pocket hotel. A crowd had gathered inside, filling the entrance and the hallway beyond. A receptionist finally led us to a small room to await the minister.

Agrawal appeared and parked his portly bulk over a chair. A young woman took a seat next to the minister. He introduced her as his daughter, a physician. The minister's office had allocated only about 15 minutes for the meeting, so Yohei kept the formalities to a minimum and cut to the chase.

"My goals here are threefold: eradicate leprosy, eliminate discrimination against persons affected by leprosy, and put an end to begging in India. You have 850 leprosy colonies in this nation. Colony members have formed a nationwide organization, National Forum India. With me today is Ghasiram Bhoi, the Chhattisgarh representative at the National Forum. He is working hard with officers of your ministry to provide former patients with medical support for leprosy's aftereffects. That includes such support as treatment for ulcers on feet and reconstructive surgery for disfigurements.

"Unfortunately, Chhattisgarh lags behind all the other states of India in tackling the task of bringing leprosy under control. Your Excellency, please lend your youthful energy to the challenge of eradicating leprosy, eliminating discrimination, and putting an end to begging. You can leverage your efforts through the National Forum. And you can receive assistance from the WHO, which I serve as a goodwill ambassador, and from the Nippon Foundation, where I am the chairman."

Yohei's entreaties earned a positive response from Agrawal.

"I am determined to position Chhattisgarh as a model of combating leprosy," he pledged. "We will work closely with Mr. Bhoi in tackling that challenge."

A colony leader who fostered economic sustainability

We traveled the next day to the Ashadeep leprosy colony, in the city of Bhilai. Our guide was Chikako Awazu, a Nippon Foundation project coordinator on secondment to the Sasakawa-India Leprosy Foundation office in New Delhi. Ashadeep was a last-minute addition to Yohei's itinerary, added at the urging of Awazu. Her work included visiting leprosy colonies throughout India and observing self-help initiatives supported by microfinancing from the Nippon Foundation. She had visited the Ashadeep colony in January 2011 and had found it to be a standout among the numerous colonies that she had inspected.

Yohei was to take part in a meeting of the Chhattisgarh Human Rights Commission at noon and in a media workshop later in the afternoon. His morning, however, was free, and he was happy to take the opportunity to get a firsthand look at such a highly recommended colony. We reached the

Ashadeep colony after an hour's drive. It stood alongside a city street across from a row of small shops. A high wall around the colony bore witness to grimmer days, but the entrance was ungated, and people were free to come and go as they pleased.

On entering the colony grounds, we encountered a group of four sculptures in front of the assembly hall. From left to right, they were a bust of Jawaharlal *Nehru*, India's first prime minister; a standing figure of Bhimrao Ramji Ambedkar, who was born into a Dalit caste and became the principal author of India's constitution, the nation's first minister of law and justice, and an ardent opponent of the caste system; a bust of Mother Teresa; and a standing figure of Mahatma Gandhi. The figure of Gandhi was shorter than its subject's actual height of nearly 163 centimeters (5 feet, four inches), and it depicted the independence leader using a cane.

As for the residences, they evinced an atmosphere that was anything but opulent. They presented a more cheerful appearance, however, than what we had seen the day before at Bramba Vihar. Each house had walls of stucco-like cement painted sky blue. Overhead power lines delivered electricity to all the homes and other buildings. The streets through the colony were broad and featured concrete pavements and ditches along both sides to carry away rainwater. We didn't see a single piece of litter anywhere on the grounds. The temperature was 42°C (108°F), but the well-kept colony evoked a comfortable ambience.

What was most appealing about Ashadeep was the sense of purpose evinced by the residents. We had come suddenly, without advance notice, so no one had turned out, of course, to welcome us to the colony, and we therefore showed ourselves around. A young woman, visible through an open window as we passed, was working at a wooden loom inside a house. We hadn't seen anyone engaged in work like that at Bramba Vihar.

The woman wore her hair in a long, neatly tended braid that hung down her back. She sported largish silver earrings and was wearing a sari of bright reddish brown. Facing in our direction on the far side of the loom, she displayed a toothy smile as she worked. A boy and girl each held a pulley mechanism that fed thread to the loom. Behind the loom, a second woman wound the thread supplied by the girl into a ball. The thread supplied by the boy went directly to the loom operated by the first woman. A second boy bided his time gazing out the window at our group while impatiently awaiting his chance to help.

"Isn't that a heartwarming scene?" observed Yohei in an admiring tone. "I also helped my mother with weaving work that she did at home when I was seven or eight. We'd enjoy chatting about this and that while she worked. I'd undo a big jumble of yarn that I held in both hands and pass a strand to my mother to wind into a ball."

Awazu told us that 16 homes at the colony had handlooms. Microfinancing from the Sasakawa-India Leprosy Foundation had funded the purchase of three of the looms, she said.

"What are you making?" asked Yohei.

"Rag mats," answered the woman who was winding thread into a ball.

The colony received orders from the state government, Awazu explained, for rag mats for student seating at schools. Each mat earned 40 rupees, and each weaver produced four mats a day.

"Where do you get the thread?" Yohei asked.

"We unravel used saris for the thread," answered the thread-winding woman. "We get orders for rag mats from people in the neighborhood, as well as from the state. People bring in old saris for us to use as raw material. In addition, the state government covers the cost of other materials."

The orders from people in the community were especially encouraging. They suggested that prejudice toward the colony residents was declining.

"How much do you earn a month from this work?"

"About 4,500 rupees."

"So we're talking about only a little more than ¥8,000 (about $100)," sighed Yohei.

"It's not much of a business, yet. But it's my pride and joy."

A building was going up behind the assembly hall. It would be a workshop for making patchwork quilts. Support from the state government was defraying part of the cost of the construction.

At another house, a woman was sorting thread out front. A man inside, who we took to be her husband, was operating a loom.

"Are you making good money?" asked Yohei of the woman in a cheery voice.

"Yes, the money is pretty good. We're making enough to save some of what we earn."

"That's fantastic."

This was the first of the countless colonies Yohei had visited where he heard of people saving money. The woman's daughter arrived home from school as her mother was talking with Yohei. She said, though, that she needed to head back to school right away for some activity.

"I'd like to hear, if you don't mind telling me, what you want to be when you grow up."

The girl flashed beautiful eyes but just showed a bashful smile and ran off without saying anything. Across the street from her house, two men were making brooms from bamboo. They told us that they bought the bamboo in Odisha, Chhattisgarh's seacoast neighbor to the east.

"Do they sell well?" asked Yohei.

"Pretty well. I took some into town to sell on my bicycle this morning and had sold four by nine o'clock," boasted one of the men.

"How much do they cost?"

"Two hundred rupees."

Yohei was glowing. This was a community where people had surely relied formerly on begging for their livelihoods. Now, they were making their way in the world through self-reliant enterprise. Something dramatic had happened to break the vicious circle of beggary and penury that was all too typical of Indian leprosy colonies. And Yohei was eager to find out what it had been.

"Where is the leader of the colony?"

One of the bamboo-rake entrepreneurs pointed to a nearby dwelling.

"His house is right over there. But he's not well," the man continued in a quieter tone. "He's in bed."

We called on the house and found an elderly, white-haired man reclining inside on a bed. This was Vishwanath Ingle, who had led the prodigious development of the Ashadeep colony. Ingle sat up and faced us, hanging his legs over the side of the bed, but his eyes were blurry, and his mind was wandering. His face was puffy beneath several days' growth of unshaven beard. We could see that he was seriously ill. Ingle's expression brightened, however, when the colony resident who was serving as our driver and guide on the grounds introduced Yohei, and he moved as if to stand.

"No, no. Just as you are."

Yohei moved over to the bed as he spoke. Bending down, he grasped Ingle's hands as both a greeting and as a means of encouraging the ailing colony leader to remain seated.

"I can't believe that you have actually come," uttered Ingle. "Thank you. Thank you! We owe everything to you. I should show you around. But as you can see, I've gotten sick. I'm sorry."

Tears welled up in Ingle's eyes as he spoke.

"You've put together an impressive colony here," praised Yohei. "I can see that you've poured your heart into this project. You have my gratitude and my profoundest respect. We'll leave you alone now and go see some more of your colony and the residents' life and work here. Please take good care of yourself."

Thus did we take our leave of Ingle without further ado.

"He looked pretty weak," Yohei observed as we left the house. "I didn't want to wear him out by staying too long."

I was determined, however, to hear more from the remarkable Ingle, so I went back to the house briefly to make an appointment to talk with him the next day. Our guide took us next to his own house. There, we found his wife working at a loom, assisted by their child.

"Each of us does weaving, and we each earn about 5,000 rupees a month from that work. My work on the side as a driver brings in a little more cash. We make enough altogether to put some aside as savings."

"You had to buy the loom, didn't you?" asked Yohei.

"Yes, a loom costs 1,200 rupees."

"How many years do the payments span?"

"Three years."

"That's incredible!"

We next met a woman who was making bamboo baskets to use as winnowers and strainers. She wrapped strands of bamboo around her toes and wove them with her hands. The woman said that she sold baskets worth 1,000 rupees a day and that her profit after subtracting the cost of the bamboo was 300 rupees.

"Of course, it varies from day to day," she acknowledged.

"Do you save any of what you make?" Yohei asked.

"I don't have all that much left after paying for the material. But I save what I can."

A musical clamor suddenly arose amid the hubbub of the marketplace on the other side of the colony wall. We were here to see the colony, however, and continued our tour. Big, black cows were sashaying down the street as if they owned the place. Several dogs were lying in the street and showed no inclination to make way for the larger beasts. A cow nonchalantly dumped a load of feces as she was stepping around one of the canines. None of the colony residents paid any attention whatsoever to the fecal output. I noticed, meanwhile, that the dung had not accumulated anywhere on the grounds. Our guide cleared up the mystery.

"The dung makes good fuel. People collect the stuff, dry it, and use it for kindling. It also makes good fertilizer."

On the other side of the street the sight of a woman making brooms from rice straw caught my eye. She had carried a load of straw home and put it down in front of her house. There, she was grasping a handful at a time, placing it on the street, rolling the stalks with a foot to spread the ends, and then wrapping red tape around the stalks below to make the handle. The brooms were just like those that were long a familiar sight at households throughout Japan. I strolled over with our guide to ask her about the work, and I learned, among other things, that she sold the brooms for 25 rupees apiece.

"This is all thanks to the man you just met," exclaimed our excellent guide. "Vishwanath is the one who made this kind of work happen here at this colony. This place was just a cemetery. Vishwanath created a colony here in 1965. He got the state government to provide meaningful work for the residents to do. He struggled hard to make this all possible."

"Why do you think that other colonies haven't been able to do the same thing?" asked Yohei.

"They didn't have Vishwanath. His leadership has been crucial."

"This is a wonderful success story. I want other colonies to emulate what you have accomplished here. You ought to offer vocational training here for residents from other colonies in Chhattisgarh. Let's work on the state government to help get something started. That could put an end to begging at all the colonies."

A bald man with a scruffy beard and a piercing gaze had approached us and was standing beside Yohei. This was Uday Thakar, a central figure at the National Forum (Association of People Affected by Leprosy). He had accompanied us since we arrived in Raipur but had uttered hardly a word the whole time. He was prone, as described below, to let others do the talking.

"What is it, Uday?" urged Yohei.

"They're already here."

"People from other colonies? Here for vocational training?"

"Yes, that's right."

"This colony," added Bhoi, "has also spawned exceptional talent internally. Two youths raised here have gone on to become doctors. Another is working as a software engineer at IBM. Yet another has earned a doctoral degree."

"That's amazing."

"And that's not all," interjected our guide. "Perfectly healthy young women come from the city outside to find husbands at this highly respected community."

Two women from Ashadeep, we also learned, had married men outside the colony.

"Unbelievable," bellowed Yohei.

"But true," confirmed Thakar. "They have truly superior people here— well mannered, diligent, and entirely worthy of the respect that they have earned beyond the colony."

"We've overcome leprosy and moved on," our guide said proudly. "That's why women look for husbands here regardless of medical history. We take seriously our role and our responsibility as members of society."

"This is stunning," marveled Yohei. "We need to get all the leprosy colonies in India up to this level. Let's do whatever it takes to make that happen. This has been a great day, an inspirational experience."

Professionalism and empathy in the battle against leprosy

Uday Thakar warrants special attention in this narrative. He had never contracted leprosy and had therefore declined to take a high-profile role at the National Forum. Dr. P. K. Gopal and other former leprosy patients, acting on a proposal by Yohei, had launched that organization in 2005 (chapter 1), and former leprosy patients filled all the official leadership posts there. Thakar concurred with that approach. He believed that the National Forum should continue to operate primarily as an organization of, by, and for persons directly affected by leprosy.

Thakar, a native of Pune, counted nine physicians among his close relatives. A maid in the employ of one of his grandfathers had been a former leprosy patient, but he didn't have an especially strong impression of her condition. He happened upon a community later in life where a nonprofit organization was caring for disabled persons. That triggered an interest in charitable work, and Thakar subsequently found his way to another such community, one where victims of leprosy were among the residents.

Thakar secured a job at the second community and ended up overseeing the financial accounting there. Some 20,000 leprosy patients and former patients were residing at 185 communities within a viable distance for Thakar to visit. He gathered basic data about the communities and spearheaded efforts to upgrade education and medical treatment for the residents. Thakar also engaged in identifying undiagnosed cases of leprosy and steering the infected individuals toward treatment.

"This was in the 1980s and 1990s—the Dark Ages for India's leprosy victims," Thakar recounted. "Families did their best to conceal members who had contracted the disease. I had some unbelievable experiences while calling on households. One family literally rolled a member afflicted with leprosy up in a rug and tried to hide him from me in the attic. Numerous victims of the disease chose to escape such treatment by leaving home or even committing suicide."

Thakar became acquainted with leading experts in leprosy, and they urged him to acquire expertise in the disease. That led him to the Gandhi Memorial Leprosy Foundation, where he underwent six months of specialized training. The training equipped him well to handle the work that he chose to tackle next: finding undiagnosed cases of leprosy, mediating treatment for the cases that he found, and providing educational and counseling support for the families of the persons afflicted. At the time of our visit, he was overseeing such work as the head of the Maharashtra branch of Hind Kusht Nivaran Sangh (the Indian Leprosy Association) and as a trustee or adviser at other leprosy organizations.

"Uday is rare among leprosy activists," lauded Awazu, "in the way he respects the integrity of those afflicted. His understanding is as much from the heart as from the head."

Thakar's preference for a behind-the-scenes role was evident in his contribution to our itinerary. Awazu had relied on his advice heavily in charting her way around India's leprosy colonies. Thakar was the reason, for example, that she had made her way to the Ashadeep colony. He refrained from expressing a judgment up front about which colonies were doing well and which weren't. He simply recommended sites that he regarded as instructive examples of the right and wrong way to address the challenges at hand and let the observers reach their own conclusions.

We all accompanied Yohei to his noon meeting with the Chhattisgarh Human Rights Commission. Typically, Thakar took a seat on the periphery and listened quietly to the proceedings. Yohei cited the UN Resolution on Elimination of Discrimination Against Persons Affected by Leprosy and Their Family Members. He introduced Bhoi, Thakar, and Awazu and explained that they would stay in touch with the commission in regard to measures for eradicating leprosy-related discrimination. Yohei also described our visit to the Ashadeep leprosy colony, whereupon Thakar addressed the gathering for the first time.

"Chairman Sasakawa has called for positioning Ashadeep as a model for leprosy colonies throughout India. That is how extremely highly he regards that colony, here in Chhattisgarh."

The chairman of the commission pledged to help with measures for positioning Ashadeep as a model colony. He noted that Chhattisgarh had 34 leprosy colonies and asked the guests to notify the commission of any problems that they might find at any of the colonies.

"We met yesterday with the state health minister," Thakar continued. "He instructed us to submit a detailed report of conditions at all 34 colonies."

Thakar made this revelation in an off-the-cuff manner, but he knew full well that it would carry immense weight with the human rights commission, a state-government organ. Sure enough, the commission chairman turned immediately to Bhoi, who was with us as president of the State Leprosy Rehabilitation Committee of Chhattisgarh, and made a request.

"Please maintain close communication with us even when Mr. Sasakawa is not visiting. Eradicating leprosy-related discrimination is our responsibility as part of our work. The state government has invested us with that responsibility, and we are eager to work with you in striving in every way possible to fulfill that responsibility."

Finding 323 new cases in a day

Yohei's appointment at the media workshop was at three o'clock in a hotel conference hall. The Leprosy Mission and the State Leprosy Rehabilitation Committee cohosted the workshop for organizations engaged in fighting leprosy and for the media. Representatives of all the anti-leprosy organizations in the state attended, and the media turnout was also large. We heard from our hosts that this was the largest gathering of its kind held in Chhattisgarh since statehood.

The participants engaged in a spirited, sometimes heated back-and-forth. A representative of a nonprofit criticized the allegedly inflated results presented by a physician at the gathering. Similarly, a former leprosy patient berated a reporter who called on members of the leprosy community present to share information about developments of interest.

"That's pretty laughable," scoffed the former patient, "coming from you, who has never paid a bit of attention to our struggle."

A turbaned man from a nonprofit voiced concern about the prospects for bringing leprosy under control in Chhattisgarh. The man raised some important issues in that regard. He noted reports, for example, of strains of leprosy bacteria that were resistant to the multidrug therapy. That brought a hush over the hall, where a lot of the participants shared that concern.

The man questioned the veracity, meanwhile, of the official figures for the number of active cases of leprosy. He stated that the official figure of 90 new cases discovered statewide in the previous year was utterly implausible and offered convincing evidence for his assertion.

"We conducted our own hunt for undiagnosed cases with help from members of the colonies that we serve. The result: 323 new cases. In one day! Obviously, lots more cases remain undetected in this state. The state government needs to put more effort into finding those people.

"I've been doing this work for five years. It has included a continuing battle against discrimination. I've learned that early detection is crucial in preventing the symptoms and aftereffects that call attention to the persons affected by leprosy. This disease has been a bane of humankind for some 3,000 years. Our job in this era is to put an end to the discrimination that it has entailed.

"Part of the reason that discrimination persists against persons affected by leprosy is that discriminatory laws remain on the books. As long as those laws remain in effect, discrimination will persist despite our best efforts to identify undiagnosed cases and to eliminate aftereffects.

"We at our organizations regard persons affected by leprosy as part of our family. That's why we visit colonies daily and provide them with needed support. It's why we get together like this to debate issues of common concern. State government bureaucrats who simply hold meetings in their state government offices will never resolve anything."

Indian states had at least 15 laws that discriminated against persons affected by leprosy at the time of our visit. Odisha's state legal code included some especially pernicious laws. Elected officials there were subject to removal from office, for instance, if they were discovered to have leprosy, mental illness, or tuberculosis. Multiple laws cited spousal leprosy as grounds for divorce.

Chhattisgarh also had a law on the books that discriminated against persons affected by leprosy. The law, which predated the partition from Madhya Pradesh, barred individuals who had "contagious leprosy" from seeking office in village elections.

Discriminatory laws of the sort found in India were a target of the UN Resolution on Elimination of Discrimination Against Persons Affected by Leprosy and Their Family Members and the accompanying set of principles and guidelines. Yohei and his kindred spirits saw the UN as a powerful ally in pushing for the abolishment of such legal obscenities.

Legal events in Odisha spurred Yohei to write in September 2008 to the chief justice of India's Supreme Court. An organization of former leprosy patients in Odisha had launched a fight against a discriminatory state law in 2008. The law in question prohibited persons afflicted by leprosy from running for office in local government elections or from holding jobs in local government agencies. It cited as the basis for that prohibition the supposed danger of the transmission of the disease. The legal fight went all the way to India's Supreme Court, which ruled against the plaintiffs.

Yohei took exception to the Supreme Court ruling and expressed his strong objection in a letter to the then chief justice, K. G. Balakrishnan. He dispatched the letter under his twin titles of WHO Goodwill Ambassador for Leprosy Elimination and as the Japanese Government Goodwill Ambassador for the Human Rights of Persons Affected by Leprosy, and he sent a copy of the letter to India's Ministry of Health and Family Welfare. Yohei made the following points in his letter:

- Leprosy is curable, and patients cannot transmit the disease to other persons after they have begun receiving pharmaceutical treatment.
- Most people will not contract leprosy even through contact with persons who have the disease in a communicable stage.
- The Supreme Court, in upholding Odisha's discriminatory law, has reinforced the stigma that prevents leprosy-affected persons from leading ordinary lives.
- This June, the 47 members of the UN Human Rights Council, including India, unanimously adopted a resolution that calls for eliminating leprosy-related discrimination.
- I call on the Supreme Court to revisit the upholding of the Odisha law and issue a ruling consistent with medical fact and with human dignity.

The Indian health ministry later dispatched a letter to the Odisha state government that called for revising the discriminatory law. It included a copy of Yohei's letter in the supporting documentation appended to the letter. The state government of Odisha formally agreed on February 21, 2012, to purge the discriminatory content from the law. Thus have UN resolutions, though not legally binding, served as valuable tools in reforming discriminatory laws.

"India's state governments have all received copies of the UN resolution and the accompanying principles and guidelines," Yohei reminded the workshop participants in his closing remarks. "They don't necessarily take the initiative, however, in acting on this input. We need to call attention to discrimination, legal or otherwise, that is inconsistent with the UN resolution. That means any unfair treatment of people who have or have had leprosy. It means any unfair treatment of their family members. If their children don't have free access to education, it means demanding that access.

"So how do we proceed? In the National Forum, we have a platform for reaching out to state government authorities. The forum is also a platform for supporting self-help initiatives at the colonies and for providing government agencies with accurate information about the colonies. Let us bear in mind that the residents at each colony possess at least a latent interest in working. But they lack opportunities.

"Take a look at the Ashadeep colony. What has happened there is proof that people given the opportunity to work will make the most of that opportunity. The people there have created a community that commands respect. Notions of prejudice that have festered over the years will give way to respect in the face of self-reliant enterprise. Friends, we have in the Ashadeep colony a showcase of overcoming prejudice. Let us propagate the lessons of that showcase throughout Chhattisgarh and throughout India."

"No more leprosy"

We set out the next morning at 6:30 to visit the Santvinoda leprosy colony in Rajim. What we found there was a sad contrast with what we had seen at the Ashadeep colony.

The Santvinoda colony was home, at the time of our visit, to 50 residents, including 15 children, in 15 households. Only elderly people were to be seen on the grounds, however, when we arrived. They bore the same blank looks of hopelessness that we had seen on the residents at the Amria leprosarium in Alexandria. A bodhi tree stood in the middle of a courtyard. For some reason, someone had plastered the trunk with cement up to a height of nearly a meter and a half.

"You'd think," Yohei muttered, "that they wouldn't have to torture a bodhi tree like that. They're all beggars here," he continued as he plopped himself down into a chair wearily, not bothering to brush away the flies that swarmed about his face. "They're all out begging." He then added after a pause, "As long as we're here, we might as well go have a look at where they do what they do."

The Santvinoda colony is on Chhattisgarh's largest river, the Mahanadi, near two consecutive confluences with tributaries.

"People long regarded confluences as divine phenomena," explained Yohei. "That's why you have a big temple nearby where worshippers come to pay their respects to the gods. And the temple is a natural place for begging.

We walked toward the temple on the right bank, making our way past cows lounging along the way. A woman who looked to be in her 60s came up a path, spread a frayed vinyl mat that was just big enough to accommodate her, and sat down. About 15 other women were already seated in similar fashion ahead of us on the approach to the temple. They informed us unhesitatingly when asked that they were from the colony. None of the faces revealed any disfigurement, but fingers and toes veered out at unnatural angles and were missing in places.

"How's business?" Yohei asked a woman of middle age.

She looked up and replied with a feeble voice and a sleepy-eyed look, "I haven't gotten anything for 10 days."

Yohei left her with an offering of alms. We wondered where the men were but didn't bother to ask.

Our next stop was a boarding school for about 400 schoolchildren, the offspring of leprosy patients and former patients. They ranged from elementary school age to high school age. Fog hung over the dung-strewn setting. The students, dressed in dark-brown uniforms, all turned out to welcome our group. A Catholic nun from Poland, seated in a wheelchair, was the principal. Yohei greeted her with a smile but looked back at me and expressed reservations about the setup.

"You've got to wonder if this is really best for the kids: bring them together here at one place, have them live here, continue it all the way through high school. That's bound to make them easy targets for discrimination when they graduate and go out into the world. I can't help thinking that the kids would be better off going to regular schools."

What we were seeing was essentially a comfortable concentration camp. The students launched into a choral chant: "No more leprosy, no more leprosy." One innocent-faced youth after another joined the swelling chorus, but the effect was somehow more chilling than gratifying. Our hosts showed us the dormitory and the health center, but Yohei had little interest in seeing anything further, and we made a swift exit.

Back in Raipur, Yohei's afternoon schedule included a press conference, a meeting with members of National Forum India, an interview with a reporter from a local newspaper, and talks with health officials. I left the group after the press conference to return to the Ashadeep colony for my appointment with Ingle. Joining me was Masato Seko, a program officer at the Sasakawa Peace Foundation.

Vishwanath Ingle

The self-reliance that Ingle had instilled in the Ashadeep colony was on display as I arrived back for our appointment. As we entered the grounds, we encountered a bustle of construction work. Six husbands and wives were hard at work erecting a two-story building on what had been a vacant lot the day before. We asked about the structure and learned that it was to be housing for some women who were about to join the colony. Two men that I recalled seeing the previous day were mixing cement on a metal sheet. Women scooped it up in buckets to carry on their heads to the construction site. A man on a ladder received the buckets from the women and hauled them up to the second floor where his coworkers applied it expertly to metal cladding.

So skillful were the workers that I concluded that they were probably builders by profession. On weekdays, they presumably ventured out from the colony to do construction work in the city. I had come on a Saturday, and they were using their day off, I guessed, to do volunteer work for the colony.

Ingle, who'd been barely able to sit up in bed the day before, was waiting in front of his house. He was sitting on the ground at the entrance, leaning on a wall. Ingle apologized for receiving us in that posture and explained, unnecessarily, that it was on account of his physical condition. I sat down beside him to talk.

"Please extend my heartfelt regards to Mr. Sasakawa," Ingle began. "We are all grateful for what he has given us. He made possible the work that people are doing here. I feel bad that I wasn't able to talk with him properly when he paid a visit yesterday."

Ingle stopped abruptly. He seemed to have something caught in his throat. His eyes were yellow and blurry. The right eye blinked periodically, but the left one remained fixedly open. His right toes were barely more than stubs. Both ankles were swollen and splayed outward. His right hand was swollen, the ring finger and little finger somewhat misshapen. I got the impression that he couldn't move his left arm, which hung limply at his side. I picked up the conversation from my end.

"You have a wonderful colony. I saw people busy building something as we entered the colony today. What are they making?"

"About thirty women who have suffered hardship have established an organization to provide mutual support. Eighteen of them want to live here so we're building a place for them to stay. The other twelve will live somewhere else. The money for the construction came from the state."

We had agreed on 30 minutes for the interview, so I shifted to the subject of my visit. I asked Ingle to tell me as much as possible of his life story in the time available. He generously spared more than the agreed-upon time, and here is a summary of what he said.

Ingle was born in 1937 in what is now the state of Maharashtra, the state of Telangana's neighbor to the west. He was born in the Amravati District city of Achalpur, at the northern end of the Deccan Plateau. Ingle was the youngest of four children, two boys and two girls, in a middle-class family. His father was a production line manager at a garment factory.

The diagnosis of leprosy came when Ingle was a 20-year-old student at a military academy. Amravati had a higher-than-average prevalence of leprosy, but Ingle was the only person in his family to have contracted the disease, and he knew of no one else in the community who had experienced the same fate. A medical inspection team discovered his disease and directed him to a leprosarium near Achalpur. That was before the development of the multidrug treatment, but Ingle received the sulfone drug dapsone, which arrested the progress of his symptoms.

Ingle taught Marathi, the official language of Maharashtra; arithmetic; and geography to fourth graders at the leprosarium school. His leprosy worsened, however, as the bacteria mutated into a dapsone-resistant strain, and he moved in 1960 to a hospital in Chhattisgarh, then part of Madhya Pradesh, for intensive treatment. Ingle had already lost movement in the little finger and ring finger on his right hand, and he lost movement in his left arm soon after entering the Chhattisgarh facility. His overall condition improved notably after a month of intensive care, but his left eye developed the lagophthalmos (eyelid stuck open) that I noticed as we talked.

Unlike most victims of leprosy in India, Ingle experienced no discrimination after his initial diagnosis, and his parents provided loving support. His first encounter with leprosy prejudice occurred when he left the Chhattisgarh hospital after a month of treatment and returned to the leprosarium near Achalpur. A man afflicted by the disease was lying prostrate on the train platform where Ingle disembarked. The other passengers simply ignored the unfortunate person, so Ingle found a police officer and sought help. They discovered on returning to the man on the platform, however, that he was dead.

Ingle stayed around long enough to ensure that the body at least got moved to a mortuary, but he resolved then and there that Achalpur was no place for someone struggling with leprosy. He returned to Chhattisgarh, where he entered a leprosarium and worked as a storekeeper. Ingle later moved to Bhilai, where he secured what he calls "a pretty good job" at a steel plant. He subsequently went into business on his own selling office supplies and furniture to the steel plant and to other companies in the city.

The business prospered, and Ingle broadened his commercial scope. He began purchasing soap and shampoo in Kolkata and Mathura to sell in leprosy colonies in Raipur. All the while, he was commuting to a leprosarium for treatment. He met there the woman who is now his wife, and the newlyweds lived in Raipur for two years. Discrimination reared its ugly head, however, in an incident that led to the founding of the Ashadeep colony.

Ingle's wife was fetching water at the neighborhood well. Some of the neighbors told her that she couldn't use the well on account of her leprosy. The Ingles even received a threatening letter. That prompted the couple to leave Raipur and move to Bhilai. Three or four persons afflicted by leprosy were living in the woods beside a desolate and dingy cemetery. Ingle gave them 20 rupees to build huts. They built five huts and, amazingly, repaid the money to Ingle when they were done. That was the beginning of today's Ashadeep colony. The year, as our guide at Ashadeep had reported, was 1965.

Other persons who had struggled with leprosy heard of the budding community and moved there. The residents were not exactly "squatters," since the cemetery was not under the ownership or management of either private or municipal interests. It was simply an abandoned plot of land where people brought bodies to cremate or bury in makeshift graves.

Ingle held classes for the residents to provide them with rudimentary education. In 1976, he organized the residents into a formal association and thereafter represented them as the colony leader. He called on the state government to recognize the members' residency rights and to make pension payments, including disability benefits, to the members. Ingle collected monthly dues of 25 paise (one fourth of a rupee) from each resident and used the proceeds to make improvements like leveling the land and installing street lights.

As the colony grew, people in the vicinity, fearful of contagion, protested its existence. The colony received an eviction order from the state government. Ingle gathered officially acknowledged scientific documentation that affirmed that leprosy was minimally contagious and posed no health risk to neighbors. He won a rescindment of the state eviction order, and he assuaged the neighbors' concerns by agreeing to build a wall, funded by the state government, around the colony.

Ingle was arrested repeatedly in the course of his activism—19 times in 1985 alone. That activism was as diverse as it was energetic: blocking a road to protest the eviction order, campaigning successfully for colony residents' right to sell their wares at a marketplace from which they had been banned, leading a 600-person demonstration in New Delhi to call for safeguarding the rights of persons affected by leprosy, holding a hunger strike during a two-month incarceration. And it was highly successful in transforming the environment for persons affected by leprosy. Witness the change in the posture of state and local governments. Official agencies that formerly treated Ingle as a pariah now invite him to come forward with ideas for addressing problems.

The Leprosy Mission has been especially supportive of Ashadeep. Advisers from that organization oversaw the creation of 20 self-help groups at the colony. And a 50,000 rupee grant from the Leprosy Mission funded an early round of construction work that put in place quality housing and basic infrastructure.

Ingle later learned of Yohei's philanthropic activity in the fight against leprosy and against leprosy-related discrimination. He was incredulous that someone in faraway Japan could have taken a proactive interest in leprosy issues in India. Putting aside his doubt, he applied through the International Leprosy Union for financial support from the Sasakawa Memorial Health Foundation, and the colony received a 200,000 rupee loan. It used the funds to build housing for single women and to purchase looms.

Education, emphasizes Ingle, is fundamental to nurturing self-reliance. He emphasizes, too, the power of faith. A devout Christian, Ingle attributes Ashadeep's success to divine oversight. His is an open and accepting faith, and Christians mingle in a friendly symbiosis with Buddhists and Hindus at the colony.

I summoned the courage to ask a difficult question before bidding Ingle farewell. Yohei had mentioned that some of India's leprosy colonies engaged in bootlegging as a source of sustenance and that the government turned a blind eye to the practice. Ingle responded to my query with silence. Our guide answered in his stead.

"Ashadeep had bootlegging, too. But this man," he said while gesturing toward Ingle, "laid down the law. He declared that it was unacceptable and put an end to the practice. We'd like to export some of the things that we make here. That could mean more than what we're making now. For example, we could make plastic dishes. We have some money in reserve that we could use to buy the necessary equipment, and we have the land for new workrooms, but we don't have enough money to build the structures. We're thinking of asking Mr. Sasakawa for some loan financing."

In his element

We flew the next day to Hyderabad. That city lay across Chhattisgarh's southern border in the Telangana region of what was then the state of Andhra Pradesh. At the time of our visit, separatists were agitating for statehood for Telangana, and the local authorities arranged a military escort to ensure our safety. Telangana did in fact become a state in 2014. Hyderabad, however, will remain the de jure capital of Andhra Pradesh, as well as the capital of Telangana, for up to 10 years.

From Hyderabad's Rajiv Gandhi International Airport, we headed directly to the press club, where Yohei was to address a media gathering. Cows were less numerous on the streets here than in Chhattisgarh, and getting around was therefore a lot easier. The media gathering was lively. A lot of journalists at the gathering would accompany Yohei on his three-day itinerary in the state, and they demonstrated a generally good grasp of the issues. Some noted, for example, the value of fostering socioeconomic self-reliance in eliminating discrimination. One called for building more rehabilitation centers for former leprosy patients.

A three-hour drive from the press club took us to the Devanagar leprosy colony, in the city of Nizamabad. We had a thoroughly enjoyable ride through woods and rice paddies. I took the opportunity to apprise Yohei of what I had heard from Ingle. The road was good, notwithstanding some occasional construction work, and we arrived without a hitch.

Devanagar occupies a setting of striking natural beauty. It was home to about 850 people in 180 households at the time of our visit. We learned that 84 of the residents were receiving treatment for leprosy, down from around 6,000 in 1985. Scores of residents turned out to greet Yohei. Joining them were the members of the media retinue and our security detail.

The leader of the colony appeared and delivered a long-winded welcome. Yohei's gaze wandered as the leader droned on. When his turn came to address the gathering, he kept the formalities short and sweet. He was eager to move on to more meaningful interaction.

"Let's get to know each other," Yohei bellowed and jumped into the crowd, dishing out handshakes and hugs and words of encouragement.

Yohei was in his element.

6

MOTHERS AND CHILDREN TORN APART
RIO DE JANEIRO

We embarked for Brazil on November 23, 2011. Nonstop flights are unavailable between Japan and Brazil, so we traveled via New York. We left Narita on the 23rd, spent a night at a hotel near John F. Kennedy International Airport, and flew the next day to São Paulo's Guarulhos International Airport.

Brazil in 2011 was the last remaining nation that had not attained the WHO's "elimination" benchmark for leprosy: less than 1 active case per 10,000 population. According to Brazilian government statistics, the prevalence rate had plummeted from 18.9 in 1990 to 4.9 in 1998 but had subsequently hovered between 4 and 5 until 2003. Some 3,521—64%— of Brazil's 5,500 officially incorporated cities, towns, and villages reported active cases as of 2002. The prevalence rate in Brazil resumed its downward trend in 2004 and had declined to 1.98 in 2007 and to 1.62 in 2011.

Part of the challenge in coming to terms with leprosy in Brazil is the unreliability of the statistics. The methodology employed by Brazil's health ministry in gathering data does not conform with the WHO's methodology. That results in a gap between the Brazilian government statistics and those prepared by the WHO. Brazil's government reported a prevalence rate of 4.17 (4.17 cases per 10,000 population) for 2002, whereas the WHO calculated the rate at 2.98.

The difference of 1.19 corresponds to 27,340 active cases. That difference is attributable to multiple factors. The Brazilian government's figures include patients who had received enough multidrug therapy (MDT) for the WHO to regard them as cured. In addition, the Brazilian government's calculations apparently include out-of-date records for former patients.

On the other hand, the figures calculated with either methodology surely understate the immensity of the problem. That's because the rainforest in Brazil's Amazon basin surely harbors countless undetected cases of leprosy.

2002

Yohei made his first visit to Brazil in January 2002 and was appalled at the government's laxity in addressing the problem of leprosy. Progress in reducing the prevalence of the disease had stalled under the administration of then President Fernando Henrique Cardoso (born 1931, president from 1995 to 2002). Yohei met in Brazil with Cardoso, who pledged to step up the leprosy-control effort, but nothing happened.

2004

Luiz Inácio Lula da Silva (popularly known as Lula; born 1945, president from 2003 to 2011) won the 2002 presidential election, and his inauguration engendered optimism about the prospects for a stepped-up government commitment to battling leprosy. Soon after taking office, Lula became the first Brazilian president in about a century to visit a leprosy care facility. He expressed a strong commitment to addressing the problem of leprosy when he met Yohei in Brasília in 2004.

"We could have solved this problem of leprosy long before, but we did not try hard enough. We need to make up for lost time."

Lula installed a new team in the health ministry to manage the leprosy-control effort. He also moved to right past wrongs. Brazil adopted a policy in 1923 that provided for committing sufferers of leprosy to isolation hospitals, and it strengthened the provisions for identifying and isolating sufferers in 1949. Isolation policy remained in effect in some Brazilian states until the 1980s. Under Lula, the government indemnified individuals who had been subjected to compulsory hospitalization on account of leprosy.

Lula was sensitive, meanwhile, to the importance of tackling the social issue of the need for eliminating leprosy-related discrimination, as well as the medical task of controlling the disease. Witness his remarks on receiving a UN award in December 2010 for his nation's HIV/AIDS program.

"As I, myself, have been a victim of prejudice for my entire life, I know the prejudice against me, I know the prejudice against the poor, against the people with leprosy, and I know the prejudice against black people in this country. I know the prejudice against women on the election campaign, and I know the prejudice against HIV-positive people. Anything I can do to help in battling prejudice, I will, because I think prejudice is the most damaging disease in humanity."

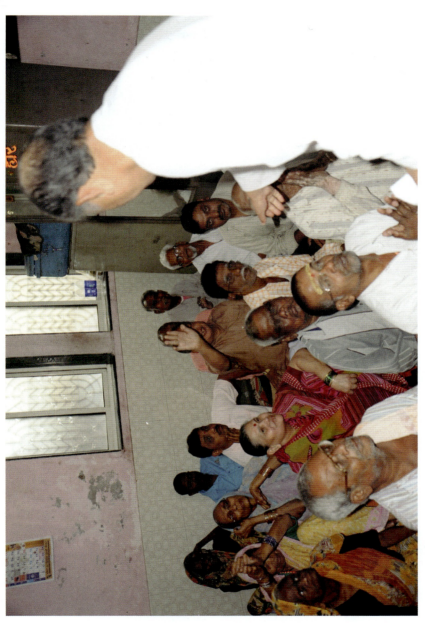

1. Yohei with residents at the Sanjay Nagar leprosy colony near Mumbai (December 2010)

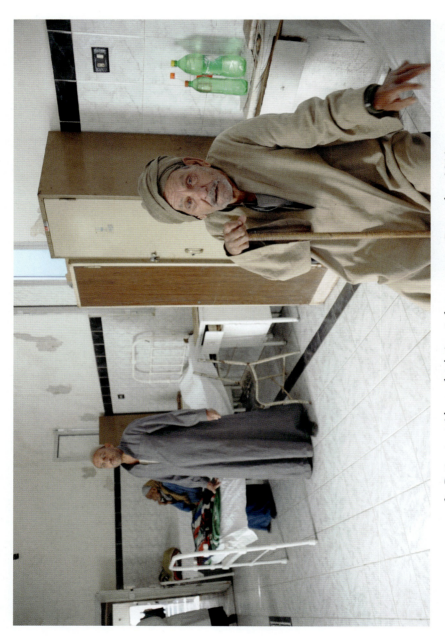

2. Patients at Alexandria's Amria leprosarium (December 2010)

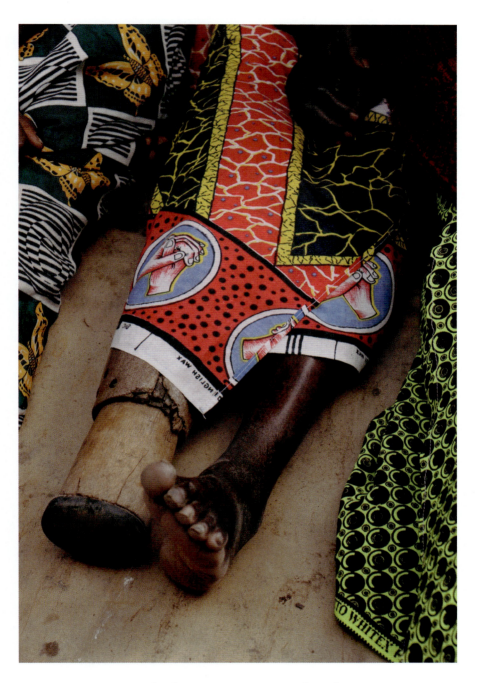

3. A wooden leg on a woman in Utale (July 2011)

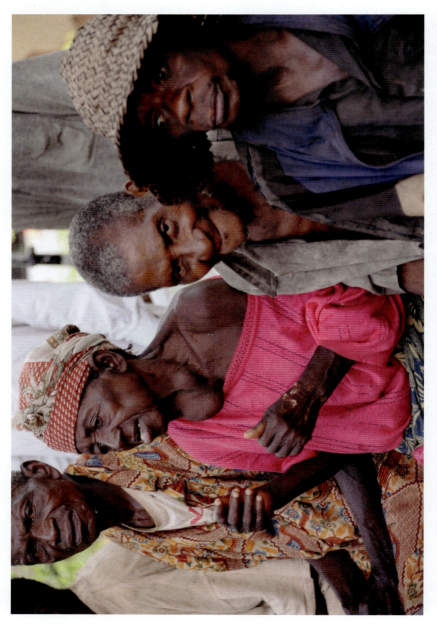

4. Leprosy patients and cured persons in the village of Kaka, Lobaye (July 2011)

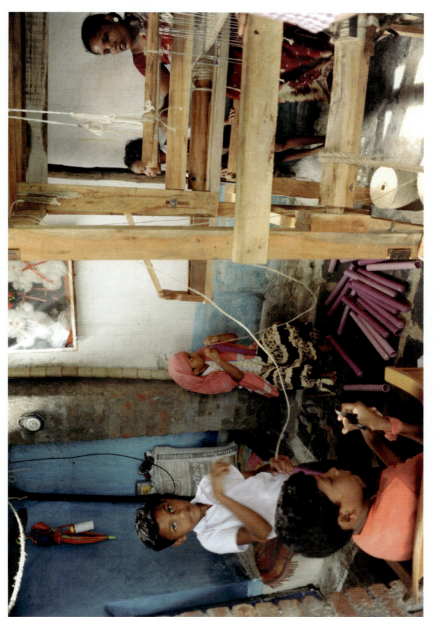

5. Self-reliance through weaving at the Ashadeep leprosy colony (September 2011)

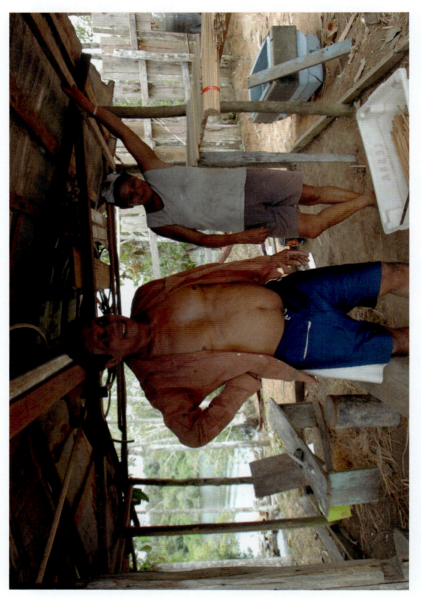

6. A husband and wife, cured leprosy patients, who have secreted themselves from society in the depths of the Amazon jungle (June 2006)

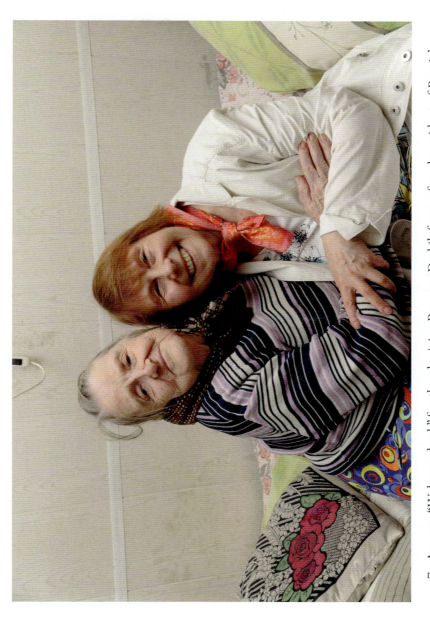

7. A warm "Welcome back" for the physician Romana Drabik from a female resident of Russia's Astrakhan leprosarium (June 2012)

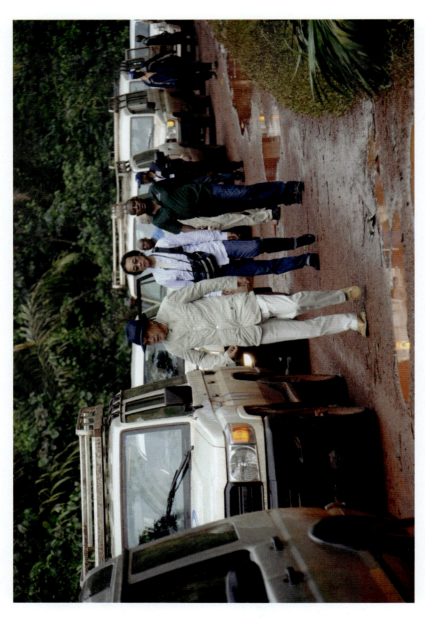

8. Yohei, the author (second in line), and other members of their party on a muddy road in the Congo, bound for a pygmy village (April 2015)

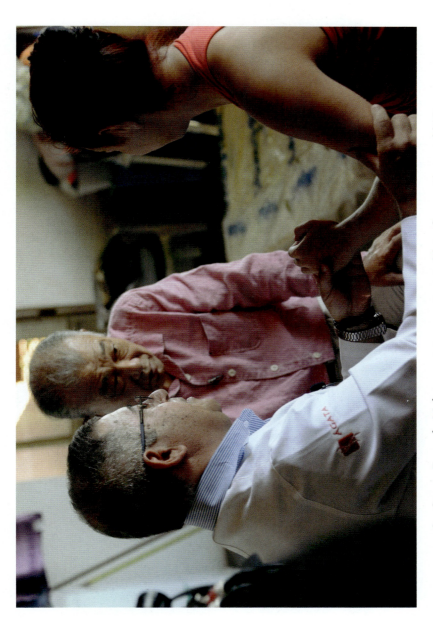

9. Cicero Frasa de Melo examining a patient in Mato Grosso (August 2015)

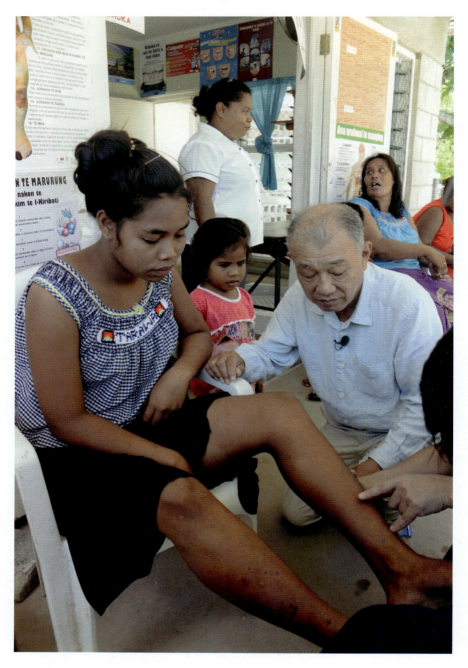

10. A sixteen-year-old girl, who has just received a diagnosis of leprosy, in Kiribati (October 2015)

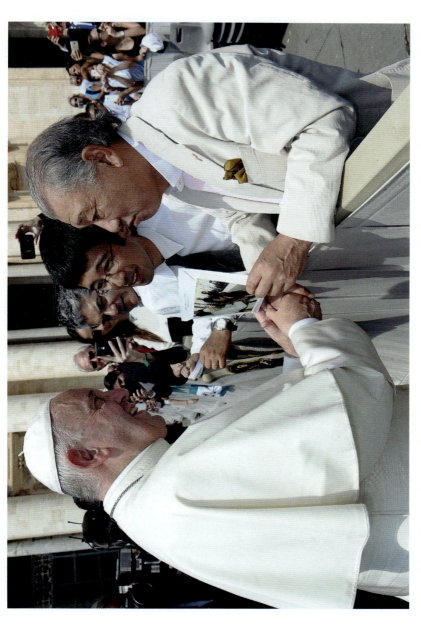

11. Yohei with two popes at the Vatican: Francis in person, John Paul II in a photo of an earlier audience (June 2016)

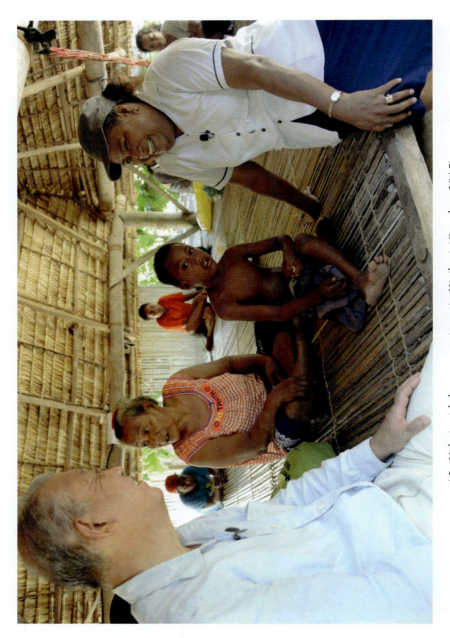

12. Yohei with leprosy patients in Kiribati (October 2015)

2005

Yohei returned to Brazil at the end of February 2005 to attend a seminar in Rio de Janeiro on leprosy and human rights. After participating in the seminar, he visited a health center in Rio and the Curupaiti leprosy colony in the nearby municipality of Nova Iguaçu. That city had the highest prevalence rate in the state of Rio de Janeiro, at around 5. The rate had reportedly spiked after Nova Iguaçu's health center closed for two years for renovation in the late 1990s and 40% of the city's registered patients stopped receiving treatment. That was a troubling tale, but it hardly accounted for the still-high prevalence rate.

Seeking answers, Yohei met with the head of the municipal department of health. The department head, who had been on the job for just two months, described a long-standing pattern of misappropriating funds and medicine. He claimed to be leading a cleanup of the department despite threats to his life, but Yohei found his account unconvincing.

2006

The task of monitoring Brazilian progress in tackling leprosy led Yohei back to the nation in June 2006. A whirlwind itinerary took him to Rio de Janeiro, Brasília, Fortaleza, and Manaus in nine days. The stops included the Tavares de Macedo leprosy colony on the outskirts of Rio de Janeiro. That colony, established by the Brazilian government in the 1930s, was home to about 250 patients and former patients. It was home to an even larger population of residents who had never contracted leprosy and who moved there for the subsidized rent and utilities. There, too, Yohei heard stories of the egregious misallocation of funds.

The stop in Brasília was for meetings with senior government officials. In the Fortaleza vicinity, Yohei visited the Antônio Diogo and Antônio Justa leprosy colonies. From Manaus, he took a boat up the Rio Negro to the Paricatuba health center in the forest town of Iranduba. That town is the site of a former leprosy sanatorium. It was home at the time of Yohei's visit to about 800 residents, largely leprosy patients and former patients and their family members.

Yohei traveled two hours further up the Rio Negro the next day. His destination was the homestead headed by a man and wife who were former leprosy patients. The couple, Antonio Motelo and Dona Maria, lived with their daughter and son and their son's wife and children. They earned a decent living by making and selling wooden skewers for cooking from wood harvested in the forest.

Antonio had experienced medical problems and sought treatment at a clinic in Manaus, where he received a diagnosis of leprosy. He subsequently received the MDT blister packs from a roving paramedic who delivered them on a regular basis. Dona Maria then came down with the disease. She elected to conceal her condition from the neighbors and to commute to Manaus to secure her MDT blister packs. Antonio and Dona Maria's daughter contracted leprosy in the wake of her parents. She, too, opted to eschew the convenience of receiving the blister packs from the roving paramedic and to commute to Manaus.

The daughter was reportedly at home when Yohei visited, but she declined to make an appearance, presumably on account of sensitivity about her disease. Yohei was astonished to learn that leprosy-related discrimination permeated even the Amazon rainforest.

"I couldn't believe that people felt obliged to conceal their leprosy in such a remote and sparsely populated setting. We had brought along a soccer ball for the kids, and seeing their innocent delight in kicking it about was inspirational. It was a stirring reminder of the work ahead of us in protecting people from disease and from discrimination."

Yohei had resolved to meet again with Lula.

2008

Brazil's health ministry was a tableau of stunning denial when Yohei returned to the capital in November 2008. He met first with Dr. Maria Leide de Oliveira, the coordinator of the ministry's leprosy-control program. Yohei struggled mightily to get de Oliveira to specify a target year for attaining the WHO's elimination benchmark for leprosy. She declined, however, to offer a clear target. Worse, she avoided even mentioning "control" in regard to the disease.

Yohei learned later from another health ministry staffer that de Oliveira had been toeing unwritten ministry policy. The tacit understanding in the ministry was that no one was to speak of targets in regard to leprosy control. That understanding ostensibly reflected the following line of thought: Even if we get the prevalence rate down to less than 1 per 10,000, we'll still get new cases. We'll be serving the people better by concentrating on equipping dermatologists and other physicians to make accurate diagnoses and to administer the MDT and provide high-quality care.

The logic sketched above, though superficially plausible, is merely a rationalization for inaction. Brazil and the other members of the World Health

Assembly, which is the WHO's decision-making body, voted in 1991 to adopt the 1/10,000 benchmark. What is more, the members voted to adopt the target year of 2000 for attaining the benchmark. The Brazilian government's subsequent backtracking was an abrogation of the responsibility it undertook in signing the original resolution.

Simply reducing the prevalence rate to less than 1/10,000 is not, of course, the goal of the anti-leprosy movement. That benchmark is just a milestone en route to the real goal of eradicating the disease completely. And truly eradicating leprosy means finding all the undiscovered cases. The ministry talk of abandoning the benchmark in favor of "concentrating...to make accurate diagnoses" strained credulity.

Brazil is one of several nations where leprosy and other tropical diseases compete for priority in the government's allocation of limited resources. That the Brazilian government has allocated higher priority to such pressing health problems as HIV/AIDS and malaria is understandable. But to put aside agreed-upon benchmarks and targets on the basis of transparent excuses is inexcusable. To sidetrack the leprosy-control effort in that manner is to condemn countless individuals to the ravages of belatedly detected or undetected leprosy.

Yohei, disgusted with the health care bureaucracy, took his case anew to the president. Lula's appointments secretary had slotted Yohei for 15 minutes with the president on the evening of November 18. Also on hand for the meeting at the official presidential residence were the health minister, José Gomes Temporão; the special secretary for human rights, Paulo de Tarso Vannuchi; the health surveillance secretary, Dr. Gerson de Oliveira Penna; de Oliveira; and representatives of Brazil's influential Movement for the Reintegration of Persons Afflicted by Hansen's disease (MORHAN).

Lula made no move to get up from his chair even after 15 minutes had elapsed, and the meeting continued for a half hour. He instructed Temporão to provide him later with an update on the leprosy-control effort and pledged to do everything possible to further the effort. The meeting yielded what seemed at the time to be two steps forward. One, leprosy joined the government's list of health care priorities for municipalities nationwide in the coming year. Two, the health ministry dispatched a directive to the municipal heads to devote stepped-up attention to leprosy control. Alas, both measures ended up as little more than lip service.

Yohei, undeterred, continuing working through different channels to press the Brazilian government to commit to attaining the elimination benchmark and to specifying a target year for attainment. His perseverance paid off in

2010, when the Brazilian government pledged at the World Health Assembly to attain the benchmark by 2015.

Although heartened by Brazil's renewed, formal commitment, Yohei remained skeptical about the government's stance. He was especially concerned about whether the commitment would survive under Dilma Rousseff, who succeeded Lula as president in 2011. Yohei sought the earliest possible opportunity to see firsthand how things were playing out under the new president. That opportunity finally took shape in our September 2011 flight to São Paulo.

2011

Our November 2011 visit to Brazil was mainly for Yohei to attend the 12th Brazilian Leprosy Congress and to hold meetings with government officials. The congress took place in the coastal resort city of Maceió. There, we heard messages of renewed commitment by the Brazilian government to fight leprosy and toured a hospital that provides rehabilitative care for former leprosy patients. We flew from Maceió to São Paulo, where Yohei met with Dr. José Luiz Gomes do Amaral, the president of the Brazilian Medical Association and the newly elected president of the World Medical Association. Also in São Paulo, Yohei stopped by a rehabilitation center and attended a gathering of former leprosy patients. The participants at the gathering discussed issues for persons affected by leprosy and progress in eliminating leprosy-related discrimination.

We flew on the morning of September 26 to Rio de Janeiro and traveled directly from the airport one and a half hours by car to Tavares de Macedo. MORHAN was holding a gathering there to mobilize support for persons who had suffered under an appalling government policy. That policy, which remained in effect until the 1970s, had provided for removing babies born to mothers afflicted by leprosy and placing them in institutions. MORHAN was working to help reunite children with their parents and siblings. Its work included analyzing records at facilities nationwide and creating a DNA database, and the growing number of reunifications had attracted extensive media coverage.

The members of the community had erected a stage in a broad plaza when we arrived before noon, and a round of entertainment was getting under way to kick off the event. Yohei, as a special guest, needed to sit in the front row for the duration. I suggested to Yohei that I use the time to interview some of the parents and children in question. He readily agreed, and our hosts promptly arranged for the interviews.

Joining me were Masato Seko, a program officer at the Sasakawa Peace Foundation; Yuko Tani, project coordinator at the Nippon Foundation; and Silvia Ruri Anyoji, our Japanese-Portuguese interpreter. Our car took us to a scenic hillside setting where homes nestled among huge trees of diverse species. Someone who stumbled unknowingly upon the lovely settlement would never guess it to be a leprosarium.

Santina

The interviews took place in the community center, a single-story, white-walled building partway up the hill. Just inside the broad entryway was a courtyard, and on the far side of the courtyard was a spacious meeting room. Despite the short notice, my first interviewee appeared soon after we arrived: an elderly woman in a wheelchair by the name of Santina.

Both of Santina's legs were missing from the knees downward, the right stump visible beneath the folds of her skirt. Her hands were misshapen, the ring finger and little finger on each folded unnaturally down against the palm. But what made an even stronger impression was her silver hair, which hung down to her waist. The face, too, was striking. This had been a beautiful woman.

Anyoji pulled her chair over beside the wheelchair and explained briefly why we had come and what we hoped to learn. Santina, who was wearing eyeglasses, smiled as if to put us at ease. She thereupon answered my questions forthrightly, retaining the smile throughout. Here is a summary of her responses.

Santina was 75 years old. She was born in a rural village in the state of Minas Gerais, which lies along the inland side of Rio de Janeiro. Santina had no recollection of her father and only the barest memories of her mother. The father abandoned his wife and only child soon after Santina was born, and the mother abandoned Santina when she was "only this big." Santina indicated the height of a small child by placing a hand down by her thigh. She survived for more than 10 years on mangoes, oranges, and other fallen and low-hanging fruit that she could gather in the forest.

A health-surveillance officer received word of Santina's hand-to-mouth existence and took her into custody. An examination revealed symptoms of leprosy. She was 16.

The health-surveillance authorities placed Santina in a leprosarium that stood on the site of the settlement where we were talking. She had sores on her legs when she entered, but they disappeared after she began receiving

119

treatment. Santina recovered fully enough for the authorities to place her with a household in the village as a housemaid. She earned the satisfaction of the family she served, and she earned the attention of a young man who made her his wife when she was 19.

A storybook turnaround was in the offing for Santina when she suffered a cruel reversal. Things took a turn for the worse when the first of her three children was born. The authorities took the baby away from her shortly after a difficult birth. That was under Brazil's draconian leprosy policy, which provided for forcibly separating babies from mothers who had suffered leprosy. She learned shortly thereafter that the baby had died.

Santina's second child, a daughter, was born healthy, but the authorities took the infant away from her to place in foster care. The mother later received a letter and an enclosed photo of the child that informed her of the girl's death at eight months. She never received a death certificate, though, and suspected that the notification was bogus.

The authorities also robbed Santina initially of her third child, a boy. Her motherly passion overcame obstacles, however, and she succeeded in retrieving him from his foster home when he was 16 months old. Santina raised her son into adulthood, but she contended along the way with a recurrence of leprosy symptoms. New skin problems occurred on her legs. Her right leg got so bad as to require amputation below the knee when she was 40, and her left leg required amputation above the knee a few years later.

Santina had thus suffered more than her fair share of sadness, but she insisted that her life with her son and husband had imparted an ample measure of joy. Her husband had remained by her side until passing away six years earlier. She reported proudly that she had two grandchildren and a great-grandchild. Her son and his wife had both contracted leprosy, and both had overcome the disease.

Brazil's policy of forcibly separating newborns from mothers afflicted by leprosy officially ended in 1976. And MORHAN has spearheaded a program of using DNA assays to reconnect parents and children torn apart under the former policy. Mustering support for that program was part of the purpose of the festival that Yohei was viewing during my interviews.

Maruni

My next interview was with Maruni, a 53-year-old married woman who displayed no outward signs of leprosy. Maruni was born in a leprosy colony to a mother afflicted by the disease. The authorities took her away from her mother at birth. They placed her in a home for infants and small children until she was 5 and then moved her to a larger facility, where the residents ranged in age from infants to teenagers. She remained there until she was 16.

The second facility had about 60 residents, all of whom had been yanked away from mothers afflicted by leprosy. Its administrators put the older children to work caring for the younger children. Maruni thus found herself at the age of 5 caring for smaller children—changing diapers, doing laundry, distributing snacks. The residents received nothing in the way of education. Maruni worked continuously during her years in the "care" of the government. She never had a doll to hold, never got to go shopping while holding hands with her mother.

The rules forbade parental visits, but Maruni's mother masqueraded as an aunt and visited her daughter frequently. The encounters took place across a glass window perforated to permit conversation, just like in a prison. Motherly kissing, hugging, or any physical contact was out of the question.

Maruni became distraught when her mother once failed to appear for what seemed an eternity and tried unsuccessfully to escape. She received a bloody beating for the attempt. Her mother once brought her a cake only to have it chopped up by the guards on the suspicion that she had hidden some forbidden item inside.

The abuse that Maruni related was painful to hear and painful for her to recall. She broke down in tears more than once during our interview.

Each resident was responsible for keeping an assigned area clean and tidy. A beating ensued when the supervisors discovered anything they deemed to be less than spick-and-span. Beatings were common. Solitary confinement was another threat that loomed over the residents.

Once, when Maruni was 15, she received some cakes to distribute to the younger kids. They were moldy, however, so she put them aside. In their stead, she found some doughnuts and sliced them into enough pieces for the children. The supervisors rewarded her thoughtfulness by forcing her to eat one of the moldy cakes, slapping her mouth repeatedly, and placing her in solitary confinement. Maruni also received solitary confinement on multiple occasions for complaining to visiting observation groups about the conditions in the facility.

Solitary confinement entailed a starvation diet, and the inmate was dependent for sustenance on friends who secretly bored a hole in the wall and passed in bits of food. The "toilet" in the solitary confinement cell was no more than a hole in the floor. Maruni described being startled by bats and mice while trying to use the toilet.

Maruni never mentioned the horrendous conditions in the facility to her mother. She had too much pride to let her mother know about her ignominious situation. Maruni received no care from the facility for the wounds that she incurred through the abuse there. She tended her cuts with rock salt, the only "balm" available to the residents.

At this point in the conversation, we learned that Maruni had an older brother who was in the same facility. The quarters for the boys and girls were separate, however, and Maruni got to see her brother only once a week, when the supervisors allowed the boys and girls to intermingle.

Maruni's mother found a family that agreed to take in the girl as a housemaid when she was 16. The arrangement provided for room and board in exchange for long hours of housekeeping work. Maruni was happy to be able to visit her mother in the leprosarium. Tempering the happiness, however, was the humiliation of having the family toss salt on her as "disinfection" when she returned.

The long work hours and the absence of any monetary compensation, meanwhile, were virtual enslavement. Maruni's indentured servitude continued until she was 26, when she finally secured a job that paid real wages. At long last, she discovered the joy of purchasing clothes and other essentials and even the occasional luxury with her hard-earned income. She also found a husband, but she declined to have children. Maruni had experienced a lifetime's worth of caring for small children when she herself was but a child, and the trauma of her ordeal in state custody dissuaded her from having children of her own.

Brazil's policy of forcibly separating children from mothers afflicted by leprosy officially ended, as noted, in 1976, and MORHAN won compensation for persons who had suffered under that policy. Maruni conceded that the compensation might come in handy as she and her husband aged, but she scoffed at the notion that it could ameliorate the pain she had endured at the hands of the government.

Nikita

The tragic tale of babies torn from leprosy-afflicted mothers continued in the next interview. Nikita, 58, had joined us during the interview with Maruni. I'd guessed from her apparent age that she was, like Santina, one of those who had been taken from their mothers at birth. She disabused me of that misimpression, however, as soon as Maruni wheeled herself out of the room and our interview began.

Nikita had given birth to a daughter in 1974 only to have the newborn torn away from her and placed in an "orphanage." That was the same facility where Maruni was being held, and Maruni, four years younger than Nikita, had cared for the latter's daughter there. The two embraced as Maruni left the room after her interview.

Feelings of numbness had prompted Nikita to seek medical attention at a public hospital. She received her leprosy diagnosis when she was three months pregnant with her daughter. That was the first time she had heard of the disease. Nikita soon found herself in a hospital on the grounds of a leprosy colony in Rio de Janeiro. She was terrified to see people who had lost fingers and limbs and even their sight to the same disease that she had.

A dearth of information from the physicians left Nikita to reach her own conclusions about her condition. She took comfort in noting that her limbs were intact, her sight fine, and her skin unblemished. Her conclusion was that leprosy manifested in different ways in different people and that the numbness she'd experienced might be the worst she'd need to face. She soon found to her dismay, however, that Brazilian government policy was more horrifying than leprosy. Nikita's daughter was born without a hitch, but the hospital staff removed the baby immediately. The mother didn't get to suckle or even so much as hold her newborn.

Someone told Nikita that she'd never live with her daughter. That was when she fully grasped the horror that she was fated to suffer under her government's demonic policy. She also began to fear that her leprosy might present a more serious threat than she had suspected. Sharing a room with her was a woman who had undergone a leg amputation just after Nikita gave birth. The woman was writhing and screaming in pain. Apart from the newly missing leg, she had misshapen hands, disfigured ears, and a dysfunctional eye. Nikita began to fear that similar symptoms were in store for her sooner or later.

A subsequent conversation with a nurse at the hospital was somewhat reassuring. The nurse noted that Nikita's leprosy had been discovered at an extremely early stage and that she benefited from the recuperative vigor of youth. Nikita would achieve a full recovery and experience no disfigurement, the nurse assured her, if she took the medicine properly.

Nikita acknowledged that the medicine had cured her leprosy and that she had only minor aftereffects. Coping with the pain inflicted by government policy had been another matter.

The nurse offered to escort Nikita to the facility where babies taken from leprosy-afflicted mothers in the vicinity were kept. Nikita jumped at the offer, of course, but was disappointed at the separation imposed at the facility. She could only view her baby several meters away on the other side of a glass window. Nikita was concerned about whether the child was getting enough milk. She was lactating heavily and wanted dearly to nurse her daughter, but the rules forbade any direct contact. Her breasts swelled painfully, and she needed to use a breast pump to extract the milk. Nikita, who had impressed me with her stouthearted demeanor, teared up briefly as she recalled discarding the milk.

She took her medicine faithfully until she was completely rid of the bacteria and posed no risk of contagion. Nikita then began saving money to prepare for caring for her child. She earned the money by doing laundry for households in the neighborhood outside the colony. Nikita's mother, too, commuted to the facility to see her granddaughter.

Hope was building, but the villainy at hand was boundless. Once, Nikita used some of her laundry earnings to buy a big doll and left it with a staff member at the facility to give to her daughter. She was dismayed to see on her next visit that the staff had substituted a smaller doll for the one she had left. When Nikita pressed for an explanation, she learned that the staff had intercepted the doll in the name of preventing infection. That was ridiculous, however, since Nikita no longer carried any leprosy bacteria. She was all but certain, meanwhile, that the staff had also eaten the cookies and cakes that she had left for her daughter.

Nikita, determined to see her daughter in person, disguised herself with a wig and eyeglasses and entered the facility under the name of one of her sisters. She introduced herself to her daughter, who was 4 years old, and swore the girl to secrecy. The ruse worked well enough for the mother and daughter to continue meeting occasionally in person until the child was 8. That was when Nikita succeeded in winning custody of her daughter.

Reunification was a joy, but the girl bore emotional scars of the hideous treatment at the facility. The staff had beaten the children frequently and had administered drugs to put them to sleep at night. Nikita's daughter required a long time to become acclimated to society. Not until adulthood was she able to interact reliably with others, and she therefore missed out on the opportunity to attend school. Nikita expressed satisfaction, however, at the life that she had managed to rebuild for herself and her child.

The daughter had married and borne a boy, who was 10 years old at the time. Nikita was a devoted grandmother, delighting in providing her grandson with the care she'd been unable to provide her daughter. She showed me a photo of a smiling, curly haired boy and proudly informed me that he played the guitar, acted in school plays, and was good at soccer.

Nikita, for all the misfortune she had suffered, spoke emphatically of the plight of leprosy victims who were less fortunate. She praised MORHAN for its work on behalf of persons affected by leprosy. Nikita was grateful, of course, for the compensation that MORHAN had won for the victims of the ill-founded government policy. But she spoke mainly of its work in helping the victims of leprosy regain their self-respect and in providing a collective voice for the leprosy colonies. She was emphatic about the work remaining to be done, such as providing care for persons rendered homeless by leprosy and eradicating both the disease and the discrimination that it occasioned.

I would have liked to hear more, but Nikita was in a hurry. She needed to go see her grandson.

Nadima

My next interviewee provided further insight into the horrors that had unfolded under Brazilian government policy. Nadima, 55, was born in Tavares de Macedo, and the authorities tore her away from her mother immediately. A vehicle was waiting outside the clinic at the colony where her mother gave birth and spirited the newborn away to a "childcare" facility in the Alcântara district of Rio de Janeiro. She spent 14 years there in the custody of sadistic monsters.

Nadima's mother had four children, and they all ended up in the same facility. She didn't get to meet Nadima until the girl was 7 years old. Their conversations took place, as in Maruni's early encounters with her mother, across a perforated glass window.

The residents apparently received a modicum of schooling, but nothing on the order of what they would have received at public schools. Work was the main order of the day from early on.

When Nadima was 8, her keepers put her in charge of caring for babies newly arrived at the facility. The sheer number of infants in her care taxed her physical capacity to the breaking point. Nadima desperately wanted to hold the babies when they cried to put them at ease, but the rules forbade such physical tenderness. Even more troubling was a repugnant chore that accompanied her responsibility for preparing the infants' formula. The administrators required Nadima to add a sleeping drug to the formula before bedtime. That was to keep the babies from crying when they soiled their diapers and to thereby reduce the burden of caring for them through the night. Protesting the practice repeatedly earned Nadima a series of beatings for her humanity.

Nadima's work responsibility shifted at the age of 9 to overseeing a room of toddlers no longer in diapers but still prone to bed-wetting. The work included washing the sheets that she collected each day in the flea- and lice-infested room. She performed the work while holding up her pants, which had no elastic band and would slip down otherwise. None of the residents had any personal clothing. They drew their garb for each day from the common lot. Nadima mustered the audacity to ask for pants that wouldn't fall down and, sure enough, received a beating for the thought.

The conditioning gradually taught Nadima to endure anything without complaint. If no proper shoes were available, she went barefoot. If important visitors came to observe the facility, she, along with the other residents, obeyed the instruction to sleep on the floor the night before. That was to ensure that the beds were neatly made in the morning for the visitors to see.

Nadima's bed was beside a drafty window, and she'd get soaking wet on rainy nights. After being awake all night crying from the discomfort, she'd take her own bedding to wash along with the babies' soiled sheets in the morning. She'd then shower, shaking herself dry, since the administrators didn't allow the residents to use towels.

Visitors would bring presents to the residents at Christmas. Nadima once received a doll bigger than her, which she loved, but her keepers took it away as soon as the visitors left. She demanded it back, for which she received, sure enough, a severe beating.

Nadima went to work in the kitchen when she was 10. She showed me a scar on her arm from an accidental cut that she got while cleaning the kitchen. It required nine stitches and landed her in the hospital for five days.

Permission to set foot outside the facility was a once-a-year event for Nadima. It coincided with visits by her mother. I would have thought that the change of scenery would have been a highlight of the year for the girl, but she said that she dreaded those days. I guessed that breathing the air outside only heightened her revulsion at the stifling atmosphere inside.

Nadima resolved when she was 14 to escape. Her mother had broached the subject at their first meeting, but the daughter was terrified of the punishment that would inevitably entail if she got caught. What precipitated her breakout was something that happened to the youngest of her siblings, then a girl of 4.

A female staff member yanked Nadima's sister aside while the little girl was standing in line for breakfast. Nadima threw herself against the staff member, protesting that such violence against small children was wrong. The woman, in response, beat both of the sisters with a stick. That evening,

Nadima made her move. She made her way through an orange grove on the edge of the facility grounds to a road. Nadima begged some change from a passerby and caught a bus. She had never ridden a bus and went the wrong way three times before finally arriving at Tavares de Macedo.

Nadima's mother was staying in a hospital at the colony and had no place to keep her daughter. The girl went to work at a household near the colony. Her treatment there was only just better than it had been at the facility she had left behind. The family kept the refrigerator locked, for example, so that she couldn't get food or even cold water on her own.

After working briefly for the family, Nadima met and moved in with a man, a former leprosy patient. That was in 1970, and the two cohabited for 24 years. A growth appeared inside Nadima's right cheek in 1991, three years before her relationship with the man ended. She went to a hospital to have it treated, where the diagnosis was early-stage leprosy. Medicine cured the disease completely, and Nadima experienced no aftereffects.

Nadima had a daughter with the man. She lacked the confidence, however, to care for a child properly and gave the baby up for adoption. The adoption took place locally, and the baby ended up with an acquaintance of Nadima's. Not until several years later did Nadima learn that the friend's adopted daughter was the girl she had borne. The daughter was 34 as we talked and two months pregnant. She and Nadima had established a good relationship, and the mother was looking forward to becoming a grandmother.

Sebastian

We saw Nadima off and prepared to head back to the MORHAN gathering to rejoin Yohei and the rest of our party. Suddenly, an elderly man in a blue-and-white-striped polo shirt appeared and asked me to hear his story. The four interviews had already consumed about three hours, and Yohei needed Anyoji for Japanese-Portuguese interpreting. I was therefore hesitant to linger any longer. But the man's eyes, magnified through the thick lenses of his glasses, were insistent.

The man's face had some pockmarks but was otherwise free of signs of leprosy. His pale skin suggested a more or less pure-blooded Iberian pedigree. He introduced himself as Sebastian Rosa Ricardo and told me that he was 83 years old.

Sebastian's father, I learned, suffered from leprosy and died before his son was born. The child and his mother led an impoverished life in a village. A sore appeared on Sebastian's face when the boy was 9. When he and his mother left it untreated for more than a year, someone in the village reported him to the local health clinic. The clinic summoned him for an examination, and health surveillance officers soon appeared at Sebastian's home to take him away. They transported the boy, then 11, in a creaking, horse-drawn wagon to the hospital at the Tavares de Macedo colony.

The boy and his mother had been close, but she never visited him at the colony. She was simply too poor to make the trip. Few of the children in the colony's hospital received visits from parents or other relatives.

Sebastian had spent all 72 years of his life since that ride in the horse-drawn wagon at the colony. He hadn't come, however, to recount the daily details of his long and lonely ordeal. Rather, he had come to tell me of the murder of his son at the colony. He hoped that I could help call attention to the crime and to its perpetrator. Sebastian lamented that the murderer was someone who was known to most of the colony residents and who had never been arrested for the crime.

The murder, according to the Sebastian, was the work of the leader of a group of residents unaffected by leprosy. Those residents had moved in to take advantage of the colony's perquisites, such as free rent and subsidized utilities. Their leader was a former policeman. Sebastian's son, 42 at the time of the crime, had been a manager at the colony hospital. The culprit, according to the bereaved father, had ordered the murder to steal the son's job.

A highly insular atmosphere had long enveloped the colony, Sebastian explained, and had provided a cover for all manner of misbehavior. The colony had become more open and transparent in recent years, he said, and crime had declined as a result.

Sebastian wrote to the minister of justice to demand the arrest of his son's murderer, but the government did not act. He later heard that the man was in police custody in Rio de Janeiro, presumably for another offense. Sebastian suspected that the criminal was enjoying a comfortable existence under the care of his former colleagues.

Before leaving, Sebastian lauded the work of MORHAN in combating discrimination against persons affected by leprosy. He credited the organization for important contributions toward restoring dignity and self-respect for patients and former patients.

False glimmers

The next stop on our Brazilian itinerary was Brasília. There, Yohei met with the WHO country representative, Dr. Diego Victoria Mejia; with the health minister, Dr. Alexandre Padilha; and with an undersecretary in the Special Secretariat for Human Rights, Ramais de Carmen Silveira. Padilha assured Yohei that leprosy control was receiving high priority under Dilma Rousseff, who assumed the presidency in January 2011. He reported that leprosy was part of a set of high-priority diseases specified by the health ministry in August 2011 and that the government had adopted the target of 2015 for eliminating leprosy as a public health problem. Brazil's states and municipalities were working in step with national policy, he added, to discover undiagnosed cases.

Yohei also heard positive messages about Brazil's leprosy-control commitment from Padilha and Oliveira. The latter expressed strong agreement with Yohei that discrimination against leprosy patients and former patients is a human rights issue and thanked him for his work on behalf of eliminating that discrimination. Padilha and Oliveira both pledged, meanwhile, to attend an event that Yohei was planning to hold the coming January in São Paulo: the launch of the 2012 edition of his Global Appeal to End Stigma and Discrimination against People Affected by Leprosy. Yohei inaugurated the Global Appeal in 2006 as an annual event for calling attention to leprosy issues. The Global Appeal takes place on or around World Leprosy Day, the last Sunday of January, and it includes seminars and other awareness-raising activities in nations worldwide.

Brazil thus flashed glimmers of promise for renewed progress in tackling the challenge of bringing leprosy under control. Sadly, that promise was fleeting.

7

A BELATED ARRIVAL FOR THE MULTIDRUG THERAPY
RUSSIA AND UKRAINE

Yohei had only been back to Japan from Brazil for about two months when he headed for Peru on January 18, 2012. That destination appeared for a frightening spell to have become Yohei's last. The alarming event occurred at Pucallpa International Airport, from where he and his colleagues were to fly back to Japan via Lima.

On the day in question, Yohei had arisen, as always, at 5 a.m., and his group had taken a one-hour flight from Lima's Jorge Chávez International Airport to Pucallpa. Their purpose was to visit the Amazónico de Yarinacocha Hospital. Ernesto "Che" Guevara (1928–1967) had visited the same hospital years before on a motorcycle tour of Peru. Yohei met there with former patients and left them with encouraging words. He then returned to the airport to begin the journey home.

"Sasakawa-san, everything's ready for us to move on to the boarding gate." Yohei failed to respond to this summons from Natsuko Tominaga, a Nippon Foundation photographer who doubled as his secretary on the road. He was gushing perspiration from his face and head as he emerged from a crouch, and he was shaking with convulsions. Yohei's eyes were closed, as if he had lost consciousness, but the gritting of his teeth suggested that, rather, he was coping with some sort of extreme pain. The interpreter, Hernán, had studied acupuncture and moxibustion in Japan on a scholarship from the Sasakawa Peace Foundation. He took Yohei's pulse and reported, "It's weak and fast."

Hernán summoned an airport nurse, who took Yohei's blood pressure. It was extremely low, at 80 over 40. The nurse brought a wheelchair and conveyed Yohei to an emergency-care room furnished with a bed. After about 10 minutes of reclining with his feet elevated, Yohei felt good enough to walk on his own power to the restroom, wipe himself off head to toe with his drenched T-shirt, and change into a dry shirt. The group somehow made its scheduled 6:30 p.m. flight for Lima.

An ambulance was waiting on the tarmac to take Yohei to a hospital, and a highly professional team was standing by there to run a battery of tests, including an electrocardiogram, a blood analysis, a CT scan, and an echocardiogram. The upshot of the test findings: Yohei had a significant atrioventricular (AV) block, and the attending physician argued for implanting a pacemaker to ensure his safety on the homeward flight. Yohei's heart specialist in Japan, reached by phone, concurred, and Yohei received a pacemaker in a surgical procedure performed the next morning.

The Volga delta

Yohei was pale when I saw him again shortly after he got back to Japan. But the experience had only heightened his determination to carry on with the anti-leprosy crusade, and he was airborne again in a matter of months.

We departed Narita International Airport at the end of June 2011. Our destination was Russia. We were bound not for a well-known urban destination, such as Moscow or Saint Petersburg, but for Astrakhan, the former capital of a medieval khanate on the Caspian Sea. Over the next two years, I would accompany Yohei to six nations in the region that the WHO administers as "Europe": Russia, Ukraine, Uzbekistan, Tajikistan, Spain, and Portugal.

Europe is one of the WHO's six administrative regions, along with Africa, the Americas, the Eastern Mediterranean, Southeast Asia, and the Western Pacific. It comprises 53 nations, and the WHO had long since stopped publishing comprehensive data about leprosy in any of those nations. The implication was that the nations in the European region had eradicated the disease—that they had gone beyond achieving the WHO's "elimination" criterion of less than 1 case per 10,000 people. Immigrants in Western Europe accounted for the extremely few instances of leprosy reported in the region.

Health officials in some of the European nations had concluded that leprosy was no longer an issue and had discarded their leprosy data. Official compilations of leprosy data were utterly lacking in the swath of territory that extends from Astrakhan across the Caucasus to Central Asia.

"I decided that I needed to see with my own eyes what was going on here," Yohei explained. "The world now has only 16 nations that have more than 1,000 active cases of leprosy. So the disease is nowhere near tuberculosis or

AIDS in magnitude, and it doesn't receive much attention in governments' prioritizing. You'll find lots of presidents and health ministers who are totally unaware of the disease."

Astrakhan is a port city of about 500,000 residents in the Volga delta. The delta is of a vastness that defies the imagination of those of us unaccustomed to such riverine immensity. Unfolding just a step outside its watery verdure is an even vaster expanse of semidesert.

The city is the terminus of Europe's longest river. Arising in hilly country northwest of Moscow, the Volga travels more than 3,500 kilometers to the Caspian Sea, in Russia's southwest. Its delta is a lacework of some 500 channels. Those flows empty into the sea across a northeast to southwest breadth of some 160 kilometers. Astrakhan occupies a point on the Volga where the river begins dividing. Its city center is about 90 kilometers north of the Caspian's edge. A mere handful of towns and villages dot the delta between Astrakhan and the sea, enveloped in swampy greenery at an elevation of 20-some meters below sea level.

Astrakhan boasts a rich heritage as a former center of khanate power and as a modern port. It was the birthplace, incidentally, of Ilya Nikolayevich Ulyanov (1831–1886), a physicist and educator who was the father of Vladimir Lenin (1870–1924). Modernization had overtaken the city swiftly and only recently. We waited a long time for our luggage at the newly built Narimanovo Airport and didn't get to our hotel until midnight. The hotel, too, was new, and tiny bars of soap were the only accoutrements in our showers.

A pungent smell suggestive of manure permeated the atmosphere when we disembarked at the airport, and that same smell hung in the cool air when I ventured out from our hotel in the morning. The sky had been clear on the previous day, and the temperature had reportedly reached 33 degrees centigrade, but rain was falling now, and the temperature had dropped 10 degrees. A towering citadel of white walls and pastel-green spires dominated the subdued cityscape, though skyscrapers under construction were visible in the distance.

We traveled after breakfast out into the verdure of the delta to the Institute of Leprosy Training and Research. That institute serves its namesake function for Russia and for the other members of the Commonwealth of Independent States (CIS). It dates as a training and research facility from 1948, and it occupies the site of a leprosarium that was built in 1896.

Yohei received a gracious welcome from the institute's director, Dr. Victor Duyko. Above the entrance hung a banner that bore the greeting in Japanese, *Irasshaimase. Ohatsu ni omenikakarimasu* (Welcome. We are pleased to meet you), and drawings of cherry blossoms. On hand, too, were leprologists from Kazakhstan, Tajikistan, Turkmenistan, and Karakalpakstan, an autonomous republic at the northwest end of Uzbekistan. They had come to attend an international conference that Duyko had organized to coincide with Yohei's visit.

Also on hand was a retired German physician, Romana Drabik, who seemed to know Duyko well and conversed with him in fluent Russian. Drabik was 75 years old and was ever ready with a smile, but she was an exacting listener when the subject was leprosy. She would unhesitatingly cut off anyone in midsentence, irrespective of the speaker's status, if she perceived an error.

Yohei informed me that we wouldn't be there but for Drabik. Kazuko Yamaguchi, who was with us as the director of the Sasakawa Memorial Health Foundation, had tracked her down on the Internet and had caught up with her in India. There, they worked out our visit.

Drabik had run a medical practice in the westerly German city of Dinslaken until retiring in 2003. Following the breakup of the Soviet Union, she and her pharmacist husband had dispatched truckloads of medicine and other material support to the three Baltic nations and to the Soviet republics of Central Asia.

The Drabiks' interest in leprosy arose in Kenya in 1976. They encountered on a beach in Mombasa a beggar hideously disfigured by the disease. Romana was appalled at the lack of care for such individuals, and she took her concern directly to the mayor's office. That was the beginning of what became a lifelong quest.

"I decided then and there," recounts Drabik, "to cast my fate with the people affected by leprosy."

Drabik and her husband raised funds through local schools and churches to purchase pharmaceuticals and other relief supplies, and they traveled throughout Africa and India to distribute the material support through leprosy care facilities. A fateful encounter in southern India—again on a beach—drew Drabik's attention to Russia. She and her husband were in the state of Tamil Nadu, at India's southern tip. They encountered there a group of medical care professionals from Latvia. Drabik, already fluent in Russian, struck up a conversation with the Latvians and heard about the problem of leprosy in what was still the Soviet Union.

Back home in Germany, Drabik gathered information from patients at her clinic from Soviet republics and moved into action after the collapse of the Soviet Union in 1991. She and her husband delivered material support to every leprosy care facility in all 15 of the former Soviet republics.

"We were bringing in large volumes of pharmaceuticals, and getting customs clearance was a recurring problem. Once, I took a patient to the customs office and said, 'We're bringing in the medicine to help people like this.' That got us the clearance," Drabik laughed.

Drabik had continued her wide-ranging travel in the fight against leprosy after her husband's death five years earlier. Her biggest accomplishment was introducing the multidrug therapy (MDT) in all 15 of the former Soviet republics. Health officials in those nations had been slow to adopt the three-drug regimen promoted by the WHO since the 1980s and had abided by single-drug therapy.

The trailblazing work by Drabik included preparing Russian-language versions of the application forms required to secure MDT blister packs from the WHO. It also included mobilizing the German Leprosy and Tuberculosis Relief Association in sponsoring international conferences and other international exchange. That exchange familiarized physicians in the former Soviet republics with international standards for leprosy care. The resultant adoption of the MDT resulted in dramatic advances in caring for leprosy patients.

I marveled at the vitality of this indefatigable woman, small of build and 75 years old. Yohei's inspection tour of leprosy care facilities in Russia and Ukraine had just begun. We would take an overland route westward to the east coast of the Black Sea. From there, we would fly to Moscow and then to Odessa. And Drabik would be our escort for the duration.

Duyko, meanwhile, gave us a tour of the Institute of Leprosy Training and Research. We passed wall-mounted photos of the faces and hands of leprosy patients at different stages of the disease, and the director stopped when we came to a display of a stuffed armadillo. "This one was born here," said Duyko of the distinctively armored creature. Armadillos are among a handful of animal species that can contract leprosy, and they are therefore useful in research on the disease.

Yohei was more interested in living humans, however, than in dead specimens. We learned that the Institute of Leprosy Training and Research still housed a sanatorium, where 20-some former patients resided. And Yohei insisted on seeing it right away. Duyko was the very picture of sincerity. Large framed, he was of a gentle demeanor, always smiling as he talked. He complied immediately with Yohei's request.

Ethnic diversity

Duyko led us through a lovely setting that included a fruit orchard, a vegetable garden, and a pond. The sanatorium residences—two-story structures painted bright blue and green—were like a scene from a fairytale. Each house had a broad porch and a broad second-floor balcony. The architecture engendered an atmosphere that was inviting even under the cloudy sky after the rain.

Some of the residents, we heard, had lived here continuously for decades, and others were there on short stays to undergo medical examinations. Occupying the first house where we stopped were two Russian sisters who were there for a short stay. They both looked about 60 and lived on monthly government stipends of 7,000 rubles (about $210).

Most of the residents that we met were of non-Russian ethnicity, reflecting Astrakhan's cosmopolitan character. The city is the site of important oil terminals, which were a target of German bombing raids in World War II. It commands a strategic position on the Volga river system, which links Volgograd, Moscow, and St. Petersburg. That positioning has attracted emigrants from far and wide, nurturing an ethnic melting pot.

A 68-year-old Armenian woman that we met at another residence was making do with a stipend comparable to that of the sisters. She initially shielded her right arm from our view with a paper flier, and we saw when she lowered her guard that the arm was shriveled. Her father, she said, had also contracted leprosy. Yohei was relieved to hear that the government in Russia covered the living expenses and medical expenses of former patients.

All the residences that we visited had the look of a four-star hotel. Beautiful silk rugs that appeared to be of Central Asian origin and striking objets d'art adorned the interiors, and the furniture was of superior work.

We met a woman, surely in her 70s, who showed off a pair of fashionable boots. "Even these were free," she smiled, probably in jest. "They'd set you back a hefty sum."

Four Yakut males were sitting on a bench in a hallway in one of the residences and chatting. Asking if they had heard of Sasakawa-san elicited an enthusiastic response from all four:

"Of course!" One of them, whose left eye had imploded, added, "He's helped us a lot." I was curious as to why members of an ethnic group from Russia's northeast had ended up here, way out west, but time did not allow for satisfying my curiosity.

We met two Kazakh males. One, 77, had worked on ships that transported fish on the Volga. The other, 80, was a former fisherman. Both had bulging muscles from their necks down their shoulders to their thick arms. I sighed

136

at the thought that each would still be plying their waterborne trade but for the ravages of leprosy. Another 77-year-old man lay on a bed by a window. He had lost both legs and didn't respond when asked about his ethnicity.

"He looks Kazakh," opined Duyko.

A somewhat younger male, whose age I neglected to ask, identified himself as Azerbaijani and as a quarter-century resident at Astrakhan. He said that he had a sister who had also contracted leprosy, that he had a wife and two children, and that he ran a business that he had established on his own.

"I've got two cars," he boasted self-assuredly. "And I have a good life."

You wouldn't expect the sanatorium administrators to authorize free housing, free medical care, and pension payments for someone capable of fending for themselves. And Yohei wore an incredulous look as he looked into the man's face.

Yohei then met with some former patients, exchanging handshakes and embracing each. He crouched down before a man who had lost both legs and caressed the abbreviated limbs while offering words of encouragement. Our interpreter was concerned that Yohei might be overtaxing his stamina and urged him to take a break, but Yohei declined. "My job," he insisted, "is to see everyone here." Thus did he make the rounds of every residence, scampering up and down the stairs before the porch of each.

"You have a wonderful environment here," praised Yohei to our hosts.

Several female residents said that life in the sanatorium had improved dramatically since Duyko's arrival.

"This place had been like a desert outpost since its establishment, but it's become an Astrakhan landmark," offered Duyko with unconcealed pride.

The idyllic setting was testimony to the change that Duyko had worked. Jewellike droplets of moisture left by the rain glistened on the lawns. Blooming flowers beamed from planters in a rainbow of hues. White lotus blossoms stood above the surface of the pond. We suddenly came upon two reminders, however, of a darker chapter in the facility's history. Standing before us was a white statue of Lenin. And beyond the statue was the dilapidated hulk of a former prison building.

Yohei stopped and stared at the structure, which he had learned of during his 2007 visit to Azerbaijan. He had traveled there to see an example of how the battle against leprosy was proceeding in the Islamic world and had toured a leprosarium in a semidesert stretch of the nation. The leprosarium director had said that his facility had no prison block but that two leprosaria in Astrakhan and near the Black Sea city of Sochi did.

Duyko told us that the grounds of what was now his institute had once covered 25 hectares. Back then, the leprosarium presumably accommodated a multiethnic population dozens of times larger than the current group of 20-some residents.

"Orchards once covered this whole area," he explained. "The patients earned a living by tending the fruit trees."

Real estate development had long since converted most of the property to residential neighborhoods, however, and the site was now "only" about 5 hectares (50,000 square meters, or 12 acres). The sprawling grounds were still impressive, and I was in awe at the thought of the former size of the facility.

We headed back toward the main research building. A bald man with whom Yohei had talked earlier approached and addressed Yohei.

"Thank you for coming all this way. You have made me truly happy. Your visit has been inspiring."

The man's farewell greeting, obviously sincere, resounded with a complexity of unspoken memories. And Yohei requited with a bearhug.

An on-camera interview with a resident

Yohei asked Duyko for permission to interview one or more residents on camera. As usual, he had persuaded his hosts to mobilize a contingent of print and broadcast reporters to cover his visit.

"Let's make the most of this opportunity," Yohei urged, "to eliminate unfounded prejudice about leprosy among the Russian people."

Duyko, true to form, was pleasant and accommodating. He arranged for Yohei to conduct an interview with a resident after lunch. But just as our lunch had broken up and we were preparing to move on to the interview, Yohei came upon some bombshell information about leprosy in Iran and in Afghanistan. Delivering the bombshells were the leprologists in attendance from Turkmenistan's leprosy center, Dr. Nara, and from Tajikistan's Republican Center of Venereal and Skin Diseases, Dr. Azizullo Kosimov.

"Ambassador Sasakawa, I've come here just to meet you," announced Nara while shaking Yohei's hand. "I travel to Iran occasionally to conduct leprosy surveys there. Do you have any interest in Iran?"

"Of course I do," replied Yohei immediately. "But we can't get into that country right now. What's going on with leprosy there?"

"Iran has 2,000 patients."

"That many?! Is that the number of officially registered cases?"

"Of course."

"Then we've got to go there."

"You can get in if you go through Turkmenistan."

"Let's stay in touch and make this happen."

Iran was a black hole in regard to leprosy data, and Yohei had long wanted to go there. Turkmenistan is on the lower east coast of the Caspian Sea and borders Iran to the southwest. Nara sounded as if he had free access to the nation, and Yohei was eager to tap that access to meet with Iranian physicians engaged in treating the disease.

Tajikistan's Kosimov reminded Yohei that his nation shared a border with Afghanistan. And he reported that numerous Afghanis afflicted by leprosy crossed the border into Tajikistan.

"That country has 60,000 registered cases."

"Sixty thousand?!"

"That's right. And they get 200 new cases a year."

"Wait a second. That's an unbelievable number. I've also been wanting to go to Afghanistan for a long time. But tell me: How do the people afflicted by the disease flow [into Tajikistan]?"

"They make their way over the steep heights of the Pamir Knot and come down into the city of Khorugh on our side of the border. We have a leprosarium in Khorugh, and it accommodates a lot of patients from Afghanistan."

The physicians that we met in Astrakhan were networking across borders. They were working valiantly to bring hope to leprosy sufferers in a politically unstable corner of the world.

"I'm definitely coming to Tajikistan," Yohei declared to Kosimov. "And I'm counting on you to show me around. Let's stay in touch."

"Nothing could be a greater honor than welcoming you to Tajikistan," assured Kosimov. "I will do everything possible to bring that about."

Yohei indeed made the trip to Tajikistan the next year. And this exchange was the first step in that journey.

The time was nearing for the on-camera interview with a resident. What ensued was a far cry, however, from what Yohei had envisioned.

We passed through a long hallway over a linoleum floor that tossed up the sun's damp rays and waited in a dimly lighted room. Some institute researchers escorted an elderly male resident into the room and seated him in a chair positioned for the interview. The television crew focused its camera on the resident, and four or five institute personnel sat immediately in front of him in the manner of a firing squad. Yohei and Duyko took seats to the side, where they could monitor the resident and the media.

"All right. Let's get started," instructed Duyko.

My heart went out to the man before the cameras. His left eye was an opaque white, his fingers disfigured. He had surely never spoken before a large group. I wondered if and how he could summon the gumption to provide brutally honest answers.

"I'm 76 years old," he began. "I received a diagnosis of this disease in May 1963 and transferred here in 1964."

The man's speech was halting, each phrase tapering off into inaudibility.

"I captained riverboats..." he continued hesitantly, "on the Volga. We had no history of this disease...in my family. I have four...loving children. We have...a dacha."

The resident turned silent. We could see that an interview was unfeasible. Duyko and his staff looked anything but eager for us to pepper the resident with questions. The man himself showed little interest in fielding questions about his 48 years at the Astrakhan facility.

"That's enough," Yohei informed the resident gently. "Thank you. I apologize for dragging you out here for this. We can see that you've been through a lot."

Yohei stood, took the former ship captain's hands in his, crouched, and, turning to the television camera, addressed the viewers.

"I have traveled the world and met with people affected by leprosy in different nations. People of Russia, please look carefully. I have shaken hands with and hugged leprosy patients and former patients around the world, and I have not contracted the disease. Here in Russia, the leprosy population has shrunk to almost nothing, thanks to excellent work by [people like] Dr. Duyko. But please know something else. We humans have committed horrible atrocities through history.

"The worst atrocity is war. We have lost countless lives through different wars. Another atrocity has been the baseless discrimination against people affected by leprosy and the erasing of those individuals from society. I have come all the way from Japan because I want you to see that such discrimination is a human atrocity, just like war."

Yohei continued on about the United Nations resolution and guidelines. I knew the spiel by heart, yet I never tired of hearing it anew. The capacity for staying on message in nation after nation, year after year, is crucial, I realized. Yohei was setting out to change the world. The story for him and for us with him was unchanging. But his audience in each nation was hearing it for the first time, and he needed to address television viewers and newspaper and magazine readers in that spirit.

I felt sorry, nonetheless, for the former ship captain. The institute staffers had used him like the stuffed armadillo that we had seen on display. He surely didn't want to face the media like this. I guessed from his manner that the staffers had coached him in advance. They had presumably cautioned him not to say anything about the facility that could be taken negatively. And he seemed afraid to say anything at all. Whatever the reasons, we could see right away that a meaningful interview was simply not going to be possible. And the poor man was surely relieved when his Japanese interviewer brought things to an early close.

The five leprologists specially invited for the day's conference assembled at 2:15 p.m. to report on leprosy in their nations and the autonomous republic. Joining them were Duyko, Astrakhan researchers, Drabik, and the team leader for the WHO's global leprosy program, Dr. Sumana Barua. Each speaker described success in keeping leprosy under control and reported that the numbers of new cases were extremely small.

Duyko approached Yohei after the conference concluded at 6 p.m. and expressed concern about the implications of the day's presentations.

"People have lost interest in leprosy in the nations [and the autonomous republic] represented here today. Recently, they haven't even bothered to keep accurate records. The authorities are moving to close the facilities that provide care for individuals who have recovered from the disease. Nearly all of the former patients are elderly. They are already few in number and will soon number zero."

The governments' policy of ending support for former patients was occasioning misrepresentation in record keeping. Individuals who had been cured were dependent on the care facilities for their room and board and needed to remain on the rolls as active cases to continue receiving that support.

"That raises the issue," Yohei replied. "We heard today that patients in Russia remain on the rolls as active cases even after they have been cured. That means that you can't tell from the data how many active cases you really have."

"Exactly," agreed Duyko. "The figure of 382 is suspect. As you know, the multidrug therapy rids patients of the bacteria in 6 to 12 months. We've got to assume that the 382 registered cases include a lot of individuals who have been cured."

An Astrakhan researcher had reported that Russia had recorded no new cases in the past three or four years and that the number of patients at the beginning of 2012 was 382.

"Everyone in the leprosaria," continued Duyko, "is over the disease. But they need to stay on the rolls for their basic sustenance."

"We need to get the WHO," nodded Yohei, "to put the data in order."

Yohei asked Barua to show him the survey findings prepared by Drabik. Those findings, which Drabik had compiled in 2010, were as follows:

Kazakhstan	590
Russia	410
Uzbekistan	410
Turkmenistan	128
Tajikistan	80
Azerbaijan	75
Ukraine	20
Kyrgyzstan	15
Estonia	13
Latvia	10

These numbers presumably consist, as noted, almost entirely of former patients, rather than active cases. A comparison of Drabik's 2010 number of 410 for Russia and the Astrakhan researcher's 2012 figure of 382 implies attrition through 28 deaths.

Village in a wasteland

We traveled the next day to Vostochnoe, a remote village about an hour's drive from Astrakhan. The semidesert terrain was of conspicuously poor drainage. This wasteland was where the Russian government had created a village in 1960 for former leprosy patients.

"People other than former patients have since moved here," explained Duyko, who had come along as our guide. "The villagers now number about 1,000, and former patients account for only 15 households."

I was astonished to hear of people unaffected by leprosy living alongside former patients in the same village. But this was hardly an upscale residential neighborhood. The cloudy sky of the previous day had given way to red-hot sunlight. Our gravel road ran between fencing pieced together with scraps of wood and stray pieces of corrugated metal. The gaps and holes in the fencing were more plentiful than the continuities, imparting the impression of abandonment. Yet visible beyond the fencing were occasional gardens, and visible beyond the encroaching weeds were the roofs of houses. Our gravel road finally approached a red-brick clinic, confirming that this was indeed an inhabited settlement.

"Each home accommodates 2 households, and the compound comprises about 10 homes," detailed Duyko. He opened the gate in the fence in front of one of the homes, and we followed him as he strode in as if entering his own abode. Awaiting us inside were four former leprosy patients.

One of the persons inside was a 76-year-old woman who unloaded on us with a host of complaints. The woman, Taeesha, lived on a government pension of 6,000 rubles (about $180) a month and could hardly afford the 5,000-ruble cost of getting a gas line connected to her residence. She relied on an outdoor spigot, meanwhile, for her drinking water.

"I'm old," Taeesha moaned, "and I can't go on living like this."

We heard that a burglar had stolen everything of value in Taeesha's house while she was on a short stay at the Astrakhan sanatorium. The thief had taken her valuables and even her basic essentials, including an iron.

The population of the village has been shrinking since the breakup of the Soviet Union," Taeesha observed tearfully. "The young people have all moved to the city. The only people left here are old folks, like me."

Taeesha's only visible aftereffects of leprosy were crooks in her index fingers. But her unsteady gait suggested problems with her legs, too. I suspected that her complaining reflected a desire to move into the Astrakhan sanatorium, and I wondered why Duyko hadn't processed an application to secure a place for her there.

A man at another house had planted and tended an impressive garden, and everything inside the home was in perfect order, from wall to wall. His residence had running water and gas through connections that he had engineered on his own. A house further on sported a lovely board fence and a high-gabled roof. The residents, a couple and their son, had remodeled a house they had been granted. Galina, the wife, knew Drabik, and they exchanged a friendly hug and rubbed their cheeks together.

"This woman had horrible bumps all over her face," said Drabik. "And just look at her now. They're all gone."

Galina showed us a photograph of her visage before she received successful medical treatment. It called to mind for me the rendering of the disfigured Saint Damien of Molokai by the famous Japanese sculptor Funakoshi Yasutake (1912–2002).

"She started with the MDT, and it restored the lovely face that you see now," smiled Drabik.

"That's amazing," marveled Yamaguchi as she stroked Galina's cheek. "I'd love to have such smooth skin."

The improvement was the most dramatic that I had ever seen in all my travels with Yohei.

I went out and over to a cow barn and petted the bovines inside. On the other side of the house, Galina's husband was hard at work in their garden. I stepped out on the garden path and saw that he was raising tomatoes, leeks, carrots, cucumbers, and other vegetables. He waved and gave me a big, Japanese-style bow when I offered praise in Japanese for his garden.

"That couple is Astrakhan's biggest success story," reflected Yohei happily in the car on the way back to our hotel.

An 11-hour bus ride

Our two-day stay in Astrakhan ended as the members of our party boarded a microbus at 8 a.m. on July 1. We filled all of the eight passenger seats, and our vehicle headed for our next destination, a leprosarium in Stavropol Krai. That region has spawned several important figures in recent Russian history. It is the birthplace of the Soviet leaders Yuri Andropov (1914–1984) and Mikhail Gorbachev (1931–) and of the Nobel Prize–winning author Alexandr Solzhenitsyn (1918–2008). The leprosarium is in the village of Tersky, and we would stay in the nearby city of Georgievsk, 500 kilometers from Astrakhan as the crow flies. Our driver estimated that the journey would take more than 10 hours, allowing for stops for toilet breaks and for lunch. Duyko was passionately determined to help make the most of Yohei's visit, and he came along as our guide.

We would be traveling across the Caucasus, a region that stretches between the Caspian Sea on the east and the Black Sea on the west. Dominating the region is the namesake mountain range, which includes several peaks that exceed 5,000 meters in elevation. The tallest, Mount Elbrus, is the highest mountain in Europe, at 5,642 meters.

The Caucasus is home to ethnic groups of famously vast diversity in language, culture, and religion. South of the Greater Caucasus Mountains is territory traditionally regarded as part of West Asia. Here, on the southern slopes, are the three independent republics of Georgia, Armenia, and Azerbaijan. On the northern slopes are the Russian federal subjects of Karachay-Cherkessia, Kabardino-Balkaria, North Ossetia-Alania, Ingushetia, restive Chechnya, and Dagestan. Stavropol Krai borders those territories on their north and west.

Our bus crossed the Volga as we pulled away from Astrakhan. We drove past wetlands of countless watery mirrors and gradually emerged onto dry pasturelands. After about an hour, we were crossing a barren landscape where not a tree was to be seen in any direction. Mirages arose in the distance under light clouds, evoking Manhattan skylines and, alternately, high mesas. We had the road almost to ourselves and took a toilet break around 10 a.m. at a rest stop beside a monument to World War II heroes. The monument was the first manmade structure we'd seen, other than the road, on this barren stretch of terrain.

While we were stretching our legs, we were startled at the sudden appearance of a hoard of bicyclists. They numbered about 80 and told us that they were all French, that their average age was 65, and that they were riding from Beijing to London.

Resuming our journey, we arrived around 11:15 a.m. at a small town, where we took another break. We had passed out of Astrakhan Oblast and were traveling through the Republic of Kalmykia. After another hour of unvariegated wasteland tableau, we arrived in the city of Elista, Kalmykia's capital. Elista is Kalmyk for "sandy," and we had seen enough desert to recognize the aptness of the name.

Awaiting us in the capital was the head of the municipal health bureau, a man of uncannily Japanese-like features. He treated us to lunch at a Chinese restaurant, where we enjoyed mutton-on-the-bone soup and pot stickers, served on a lazy Susan, and butter tea. The soup was deceptively simple. Its only ingredients besides the mutton were salt and pepper and an abundant topping of raw onions and coriander, but the result was intriguingly delicious.

The Kalmyks, who gave their name to the republic, are of Mongolian extraction, which explains our repast of mutton soup. We had "met" Lenin's father in Astrakhan, and we had been surprised to learn that the paternal grandmother of the leader of the Russian revolution was a Kalmyk.

The Kalmyks adopted Tibetan Buddhism in the early 17th century, and their namesake republic is the only administrative territory in Europe where Buddhism is the predominant religion. Standing in the center of Elista is the Golden Abode of the Buddha Shakyamuni, a temple completed in 2005. We paid our respects there among local worshippers who, like our luncheon host, would easily have passed for Japanese.

Our road turned southward at Elista. We were now passing wheat fields, which were a welcome change from the earlier desert. The scale remained immense, however, and the atmosphere somehow unwelcoming. We didn't see any farmers in the fields or any vehicles on the road or even any buildings except, finally, a single shed. I had pretty much abandoned hope of any respite from the scenic monotony when we came upon a sea of yellow: sunflowers! The scale, again, was immense, but the floral embrace under the now heavily clouded sky was refreshing.

I asked the driver through our interpreter how much further we had to go, and he replied that we'd be there in about 40 minutes. I was a little sad at the thought that we'd soon bid farewell to the sunflowers. So I turned to Yohei in the seat behind me and relayed the news that we would soon arrive and asked if we could stop for a bit in the pleasant floral setting.

Yohei is averse to taking any detours while on inspection visits to different nations. He even declines hosts' offers to show him around when government officials cancel meetings at the last minute and gaps open in his schedule.

"I'm here for leprosy-control work," he'll say curtly, "not for sightseeing."

This time, however, was different.

"Let's have a look," he responded happily.

Yohei instructed the driver to stop the bus, and he and I got out and enjoyed strolling in a field of sunflowers for a few minutes. The sunflower scenery persisted on both sides of the road for a while after we started out anew. It gave way in time to more wheat fields and then to forest. We emerged from the forest on crossing a pass after climbing a long, gentle grade, and Geogievsk appeared below under the still-heavy cloud cover.

"It's a shame," murmured Yohei. "We'd have a great view of the Caucasus Mountains if not for the clouds."

Yohei, when he was a university student, had been a member of the university's hiking and camping club and had fond memories of his time in the mountains.

The bus pulled into our hotel at 7:20 p.m. We'd been on the road for more than 11 hours.

Caucasus melancholy

Tersky's leprosarium, which dates from 1897, occupies a beautiful wooded setting. At the time of our visit, it housed 51 residents, whose average age was 71, and employed fully 45 staff members—a ratio of staff to residents extremely high by global standards.

Yohei delivered his customary greeting to the director, Dr. Mikhail Gridasov Ivanowic, and to the staff members on hand to welcome him to the facility and then visited homes and rooms of residents. As in Astrakhan, most of the residents were of non-Russian ethnicity, notably Armenian, Azerbaijani, and Kazakh.

146

The longest-tenured resident was an elderly Armenian man who had entered the facility in 1946. His 66 years there thus spanned the entire postwar history of the leprosarium. He had contracted leprosy while living in Irkutsk, on the coast of Lake Baikal, and had made his way to Tersky for treatment. Irkutsk is on the Trans-Siberian Railway, and the man would have made the journey by grueling train passage.

I supposed that Armenia had no hospitals or physicians equipped or trained to treat leprosy patients. This facility was presumably the closest source of care to his homeland, albeit on the opposite side of the Caucasus Mountains. The man exhibited horrible aftereffects, as we had seen repeatedly in patients who had long leprosy histories. His right eye was gone, and his left eyelid wouldn't close. He told us that he had lost a younger sister to the disease.

We were surprised to meet among the residents a Spaniard. A native of Alcantara, he had contracted leprosy while working in Odessa. The man looked to be around 70 and was of solid build but had lost all 10 fingers. He identified himself as Vladimir, and we assumed that he had assumed that name after moving to Russia, but we didn't get the opportunity to ask. Vladimir was taciturn and disinclined to discourse on matters personal. With him as we talked was his wife, Alexandra, and their story cast a glaring light on the problem of leprosy in Russia.

What emerged gradually through our conversation was that Vladimir had been married while living in Odessa, that he had separated from his wife on account of his disease, and that he had met and married Alexandra after moving to the leprosarium. Alexandra, helpfully, was more forthcoming with information than her spouse. We heard from her that she was 72, that she had contracted leprosy and entered the Tersky facility in 1956, that her husband had died while she was in the leprosarium, that she had three children and three grandchildren from her marriage with him, that she had met and married Vladimir there 19 years earlier, and that she received a monthly pension of 10,000 rubles (about $300) from the government.

"One of my grandchildren," she smiled proudly, "is a law student at Astrakhan State University. And I want to get out of here as soon as possible."

Alexandra had no aftereffects so conspicuous as to draw attention from passersby on the street in the outside world. Her face showed some minor lesions, but she masked them effectively with cosmetics, and her hands and arms appeared normal.

"Do you want to live with your grandchild when he or she graduates?" asked Yohei.

"I don't know if I'll live with my grandchild," answered Alexandra emphatically. "But I want to get out of here as soon as possible and live with ordinary people in society."

"You have everything here that you could ever need, interjected Ivanowic. "Why would you want to leave."

The director segued into a detailing of the virtues of his facility. Yohei just scowled silently, his gaze averted from Ivanowic, his arms folded across his chest.

"Could she leave," asked Yamaguchi, "if she insisted?"

"Yes, of course," assured Ivanowic. "But where would she go?"

"Back to her family?"

"That's not as easy as it sounds. Discrimination would occur in the neighborhood."

"So are you basically against returning former patients to society?"

"I'm not saying that," retorted Ivanowic after a moment's pause. "This is a facility for providing treatment to individuals who have been diagnosed with leprosy. We provide the multidrug therapy, which the patients receive for at least three months. And if they show no symptoms after six months, they are free to leave. We return the patients to society. We teach them that they are no different from other members of society. We help them reaffirm their human dignity."

I got the impression that the director, his protestation notwithstanding, didn't want to turn loose Alexandra or any other patient. Yohei turned to me during the exchange between Ivanowic and Yamaguchi and murmured our shared concern in Japanese.

"This is a jail in all but name. The physicians don't want to let go of the patients. They ought to be working to return the patients to society, but they want to keep the residents here as their wards."

The back-and-forth between Yamaguchi and Ivanowic continued as we moved on. Yamaguchi heard from the director that mental care was the only supplementary medical treatment available at the leprosarium. That triggered a question as to how residents obtained orthopedic, gastrointestinal, cardiovascular, and other care. Ivanowic replied that the residents needed to go elsewhere for such care, and he acknowledged that he and his staff struggled to provide suitable treatment for the aftereffects of leprosy.

"Our biggest issue right now," confided Ivanowic, "is rehabilitation. For example, prosthetic arms and legs can become a bad fit as the users' bodies change over the years. We order new ones from Turkey, but the users require rehabilitative assistance to get used to the new prostheses."

"Let me get something straight," persisted Yamaguchi, "You referred a moment ago to '400 leprosy patients.' Do I understand that correctly to mean 400 all across Russia, including Siberia?"

"That's right."

"Are you confident that Russia doesn't have any other citizens who have contracted the disease [and are going untreated]?"

"Russians are becoming increasingly mobile," replied Ivanowic. Yamaguchi's probing had discomfited the director, but he regrouped. "We haven't admitted any new cases here for three years. Our last new case came to us in 2009, a person from Stavropol Krai."

Ivanowic eventually conceded that his biggest concern was keeping his sanatorium relevant.

"I need to find ways to make this facility accessible and useful for the community at large."

The leprosarium's population was declining irreversibly through attrition, both mortality and, as expressed by Alexandra, residents' mounting interest in returning to society. That threatened to render the facility obsolete.

"Yes, repositioning the leprosarium as a platform for providing a broad range of care is an excellent idea," agreed Yohei. "That will occasion interaction for members of the community with former patients here, which will help lessen prejudice and discrimination."

Yohei mentioned World Leprosy Day, of which Ivanowic was unaware. Activists in the fight against leprosy and against leprosy-related discrimination observe that day each year on the last Sunday of January. Yohei has staged a World Leprosy Day appeal annually since 2006 to spur renewed effort in the global struggle to end discrimination. He handed Ivanowic a pamphlet that outlined the appeal and urged the director to adopt a broad perspective and to be alert to new possibilities.

A show trial

We departed after an early lunch for the city of Krasnodar, 500 kilometers to the west, and arrived there at 7 p.m. after seven and a half hours on the road. Duyko had remained with us for this next leg of our journey. The next morning, we traveled from our hotel to the Abinsky leprosarium, which has been in operation since 1905.

Yohei had asked in advance for the leprosarium administrators to arrange an interview with a long-term resident, and they had agreed to that request. The result, however, was so disastrous as to cast the Astrakhan fiasco, in contrast, as a sterling success.

Five or six physicians faced off against a 72-year-old woman, Yekaterina. She was, as requested, a former patient, but the physicians interrupted as she tried to tell her story.

"You know that's not true!" they shouted accusingly. Yekaterina's keepers had interrupted her like that at least three times before she had talked for even three minutes. Interruptions aside, her speech was so halting as to keep us on edge, and we found ourselves wondering if she didn't perhaps suffer from dementia.

The physicians, to be sure, had good reason for wanting to manage the accuracy of Yekaterina's output. She told us, for example, that she was born in a village near the leprosarium and that a routine medical checkup had discovered leprosy when she was eight years old. That was hard to accept at face value. Medical checkups would have been anything but routine in the Northern Caucasus 64 years earlier.

Drabik, who had retained her trademark smile throughout our extended travel, leaned over and spoke into Yohei's ear in English under the shouting.

"I was here in 1995," she said, "and I met this woman at that time. She is a former schoolteacher, so she has lived in the outside world. As I recall, she has a son who works here."

We wondered all the more whether Yekaterina was indeed suffering from dementia or whether she might be intentionally uttering nonsense as a show of defiance to her oppressors. All told, the former seemed the more likely.

The director of the Abinsky leprosarium was sitting next to Yohei, right in front of me. He decided that he had heard enough and, leaping out of his seat, began verbally accosting Yekaterina. Thrusting his finger at her, he accusingly named the village where she was born and raised and the place where she received a diagnosis of leprosy. Neither place-name meshed with the geography of Yekaterina's telling. That set off a renewed commotion among the physicians, who each proffered their own "she did this, she did that" contributions. The scene deteriorated into a cacophony of male shouting. I was grateful for the presence of the TV cameras and reporters, which surely acted as a restraining influence.

"This is a show trial, not an interview," Yohei growled to Yamaguchi. "Actually, it's not even that. They just go on like that and don't even put on a show of letting us ask anything."

When in Russia, I thought, and wished that we had the time to go drinking with these physicians. I guessed that the volume would go up another notch after a little vodka and that the conversation would become even less inhibited.

Yekaterina, meanwhile, had assumed a vacant look as if she had no idea who or what the commotion was all about. She showed no sign, for that matter, of sensing the commotion at all.

"Looks like dementia, for sure," surmised Yohei worriedly.

If we were right, that meant that the physicians had failed to detect a fundamental change in their patient. The problem might be that dementia lay outside the scope of their expertise. On the other hand, it might be that they simply didn't care.

"A jail in all but name." Yohei's comment the previous day at the Tersky leprosarium echoed hauntingly. Yohei wandered off to visit other residents, and the physicians followed along en masse. All of the residents were elderly, a lot of them from Belarus and Uzbekistan. They were guarded in the face of the onslaught of the television crew and physicians and were unresponsive to Yohei's determined attempts at conversation. The television director asked no questions of Yohei or of the residents. He remained glum and silent as if he had come to a funeral.

In the garden was a silver-painted statue of Lenin. Standing in the green shade of tall, handsome trees, the statue asserted a resilience for Russia's Communist revolution.

Yohei suggested to the leprosarium director that he ought to open the facility to the community as a general-purpose clinic. The director demurred, however, explaining that his facility had a mandate to focus on treating leprosy. Yohei persisted, citing the global trend toward opening leprosaria to the community and noting the value of community engagement in mitigating the stigma associated with leprosy. The director, unmoved, simply said bluntly, "It's the law."

The Abinsky leprosarium, we had learned, had a staff of fully 131 to serve a resident population of just 41 persons. We learned, too, that all of the residents were persons who had been cured of leprosy.

"That's unbelievable staffing, incredible," marveled Yamaguchi.

"They even have a dentist," observed Yohei with a tone of resignation. "They really ought to open things up to the community."

"I learned a lot yesterday and today," Yohei said to me when we were back on the bus. "This is a big world, full of surprises. I've never seen a sanatorium like this before. A staff of 131 for 41 residents! A personnel budget to cover 3 staff members per resident. Never seen anything like it. You've got bureaucrats from the central government who are feasting here on former leprosy patients."

A beacon in Ukraine

Yohei and the rest of us in the observation group headed to Moscow that evening and flew the next day, July 4, to the Black Sea port of Odessa. We then took a one-and-a-half-hour drive to Ukraine's only leprosarium, a national government—run facility in the district of Kutschurgan.

The Kutschurgan leprosarium occupies a wooded setting and has the look of a university campus. It housed 12 former patients at the time of our visit, all of them elderly and all of them from Kazakhstan, Uzbekistan, and other homelands outside Ukraine.

Our first encounter on disembarking at the facility was with an 80-year-old female resident, Maria. Standing in front of her house and leaning on a cane, she addressed Yohei tearfully.

"The tsunami in Japan was horrible. I saw scenes of the tsunami on television and prayed to God. 'Lord,' I prayed, 'all people are children of God, so please help the people of Japan.'"

Yohei was speechless. Here was a woman who had surely lived her life amid unspeakable loneliness and despair. Yet she was praying for the victims of a disaster in a distant land to which she had no direct connection. The leprosarium directors had also expressed sorrow at the human toll of the Great East Japan Earthquake. And each had asked us to let the survivors know that people here in this faraway place were praying for their well-being.

We were amid a people of passion! I gleaned from Maria's words a visceral sense that the residents regarded Yohei as an emissary from on high. Here was a man, indeed, who had spearheaded the free distribution of multidrug therapy kits for leprosy around the world. Patients who received the MDT care belatedly might suffer from visible aftereffects, but they would be free, nonetheless, of the onerous disease and safe from any further of its ravages.

Although the WHO has recommended the MDT since 1981 and has distributed MDT blister packs free of charge since 1995, the MDT did not arrive in Ukraine until 1997. Ukraine, of course, was part of the Soviet Union and, after the collapse of the latter, became a core member of its successor, the Commonwealth of Independent States. The Soviet-era insularity persisted, tragically, in an unreceptive stance vis-à-vis medical information and assistance.

That the MDT arrived in Ukraine at all was the result not of an enlightened opening to the world but through the virtual smuggling by the indefatigable Drabiks. Romana and her husband first appeared in Kutschurgan in 1982. Their evangelizing had instigated the construction of new family and individual units by 1989. And they spearheaded the adoption of the MDT in 1997.

The leprosarium's director, Dr. Vladimir Feodovich Naumov, was thin and sported a long, goat-like beard. He had the look of a researcher who had just stepped out of a laboratory. Naumov, though, was a compassionate caregiver and a passionate crusader in the fight against leprosy. He was an attentive listener and responded forthrightly to Yohei's frank questioning. With him was Kutschurgan's deputy director, Dr. Yuriy Rybak.

Naumov and Rybak provided us with an orientation of the leprosarium. The facility was younger than the Astrakhan, Tersky, and Abinsky facilities, having been in operation only since 1945. An Odessa-born ophthalmologist became concerned about the leprosy cases that he encountered among his patients and established the sanatorium to provide specialized care.

Leprosy frequently manifests in eye problems, and the ophthalmologist had witnessed the onset of the disease early in his career in Samarkand, Uzbekistan. He was thus familiar with leprosy's ophthalmological symptoms and became alarmed on seeing them repeatedly in Ukraine. The ophthalmologist had since become a member of the Supreme Soviet and was therefore able to mobilize the Ministry of Health in establishing a leprosarium.

Kutschurgan had been home to a large ethnic-German community for two centuries. Most of the members of that community fled after the German defeat in World War II, leaving empty homes behind. The newly established leprosarium absorbed some of those homes as housing for its residents. Naumov and Rybak reported that the facility had treated a total of about 300 patients since its establishment.

A 40-year-old male admitted in 2004 was the last new case of leprosy handled by the facility. At the time of our visit, the leprosarium accommodated 12 residents—7 men and 5 women—and was providing care for 5 outpatients. All of the "patients," of course, were free of the disease and were receiving follow-up treatment for aftereffects. As in Russia, everyone ever diagnosed with leprosy remained on the rolls of the infected in perpetuity. Ukraine's official records reported 17 patients, but none of those individuals harbored any leprosy bacteria. The role of the Drabiks in promoting rational leprosy care at the Kutschurgan leprosarium became clear in the interchange between Yohei and Naumov.

"You administered the MDT to the patient admitted in 2004, right?" asked Yohei.

"Of course."

"How did you secure the medicine?"

"Through her," answered Naumov. He smiled at Drabik, two seats removed. "We started with the MDT in 1997, and that was due to her efforts."

Yohei turned his gaze to Drabik, who smiled and summarized her Ukrainian breakthrough for those of us seated around the table.

"The Ukrainians didn't know anything, didn't even know of the existence of the MDT. I put some MDT blister packs in my pocket and cleared customs at Odessa International Airport. Then I came here and gave the packs to two patients to begin their treatment. It cured both of them; healed them completely. Later, I simply declared the MDT kits at customs and didn't get into any trouble."

This woman, in other words, had accomplished alone what Ukraine's Ministry of Healthcare and the WHO should have done and could have done but didn't. Yohei, looking incredulous, turned to Naumov.

"The WHO has a country office in Ukraine. Didn't you ever hear from them about the new treatment?"

Naumov shook his head.

"Does that mean that the WHO didn't know that this leprosarium was here?"

"They didn't know."

"I guess…I guess that would explain things."

Yohei's expression betrayed a sense of personal responsibility for the lack of awareness at the WHO's European headquarters. He recovered his momentum, however, and returned to his core interest.

"And you now have no active cases here?"

"That's right," answered Naumov confidently. "None. And the former patients here regard this place as their home. This is a sanctuary for human rights."

"Do you think that new cases of leprosy could occur in Ukraine?"

"It's hard to say. Obviously, a sudden occurrence is always possible. Our last new case here, a man we admitted in 2004, had contracted the disease 20 years earlier. He had been interacting with other people all that time, so that's a concern, especially considering the long incubation period."

"How did your patients learn of this facility?"

"Ukraine comprises 27 regions. All of the regions have state-run skin clinics, and at least one clinic in each region has a dermatologist on hand who has had leprosy training. Those clinics give us a nationwide network for controlling the disease. That includes serving a lot of patients who have come from Central Asia."

"How much funding do you get each year from the government?"

"Two million five hundred thousand hryvni. That's ample for our needs."

"How many staff members do you have?"

"Forty-three."

Yohei asked the Nippon Foundation staffers for a currency conversion. The figure of 2,500,000 hryvni worked out at the time to a little more than $300,000, which was around ¥25 million. That appeared to satisfy Yohei.

Naumov told us that he had worked as a surgeon early in his career. He was working at a hospital in a village about five kilometers from the leprosarium. There, he received a sudden request from the then director of the leprosarium to come perform surgery on a patient. Naumov complied with the request and started to visit occasionally. His interchange with the leprosy patients inspired in him a desire to help them, and he ended up working at the leprosarium.

"I've been here now for 43 years. Leprosy used to be an extremely vexing disease. The patients' immunity would decline, so they'd get all sorts of complications—asthma, blindness, ulcers, whatever. We had a patient who had an ulcerated throat that required a tracheotomy. We had severe facial deformities. We had fingerless patients. We don't see that sort of stuff anymore."

"The elimination of leprosy in Ukraine is a tribute to your work here," praised Yohei.

"I'd attribute it to the skin clinics doing their job well. The patient we got in 2004 came and knocked on my door. 'Doctor,' he begged. 'You've got to help me.' I told him at first to go to the general hospital down the road. But I soon realized that he had in fact come to the right place. 'Doctor, I've got leprosy,' the man insisted. I learned that he had come after receiving a diagnosis of leprosy from a dermatologist at a skin clinic."

Naumov turned to the ethnic composition of the leprosarium's patients. It was similar to what we'd seen at the other four sites on our visit.

"We mentioned that this facility has treated about 300 patients over the years. Well, hardly any of those patients have been Ukrainian. Nearly all of them have been from Kazakhstan, Uzbekistan, and other Central Asian nations, together with a sprinkling of Koreans."

A Korean father-and-son tragedy

Yohei wrapped up the discussion with a question about Naumov's most memorable patient. The director responded immediately with a sad tale of a Korean father and son, placing on the table a business card that he'd had in his hand throughout the discussion.

"It's been more than 10 years now. He was from South Korea. He came and checked himself in here. He was missing a leg. He claimed that he'd been shot, but he had other problems that were pretty serious and were clearly symptoms of leprosy. One day, the man's son showed up. He'd made his way here from Kazakhstan. No one knows why he came. He was only about 16. And the day after his arrival, he turned up dead, apparently a murder victim.

"All hell broke loose. A police investigation led to the arrest of the father. I was aghast and protested to the police that the man was too weak to have killed anyone. They didn't listen, however, and a court convicted the father of the murder and sentenced him to seven years in prison.

"I took food to the man in prison and tried to help him as much as possible. He got out after six years and came back to the leprosarium. He'd converted to Christianity and apparently planned to pass his remaining days in prayer. But his remaining days proved few. He died of tuberculosis shortly after his return."

I guessed that the authorities saw that the man had leprosy and tuberculosis and dumped him back on the sanatorium to be rid of him. The tragedy of the Korean father and son was a haunting memory for Naumov.

"It's a really strange case. It remains a mystery."

"I wonder what brought the son from Kazakhstan," mused Yohei. "Could the father have killed his son out of fear that the boy would come down with leprosy?"

"I can't deny the possibility."

"What did you do with their remains?"

"We have a cemetery on the edge of the leprosarium grounds. Both of them are resting there."

"So you have buried other deceased patients here?"

"Yes. A lot of the patients have no one to care for their remains. They stay here."

"Here in the ground."

Rybak and a female nurse escorted us to the cemetery. We walked along a neatly paved lane that took us out past the leprosarium buildings. Turning off on a scenic path, we passed through a meadow to the gravesites, bounded by shrubbery. The graves were numerous. Some were quite old, and weeds had partially hidden some of the markers. The newer graves, in the foreground, were kempt, and things were easy to make out. Visitors had left flowers on some of the graves.

The headstone on the grave that we sought featured no cross. It was a granite slab, the top of which angled sharply upward to the right. Someone had hung a wreath of blue delphiniums, still fresh, on the headstone, which bore the visage of the Korean father. I looked at the engraved numerals, 1945–2005, and pondered the man's life. He had gotten arrested soon after entering the leprosarium in 1999 and had died at age 60. That his son had traveled to Ukraine from Kazakhstan suggests that the father had also been living there.

Kazakhstan was bereft of facilities for treating leprosy, and the father might well have learned of the Kutschurgan leprosarium and traveled to Ukraine to seek treatment. But if he had learned of the leprosarium in Kutschurgan, he would have also learned of the one in Astrakhan. And he would have traveled near the latter in passing over the north end of the Caspian Sea and across Russian territory to reach Ukraine. I struggled to comprehend why he would have bypassed Astrakhan and crossed the Caucasus Mountains to reach Kutschurgan, just shy of the Black Sea.

The thought occurred that the man might have intentionally been putting as much distance as possible between him and his home, that he might have abandoned his family and possessions, that he might have been fleeing the law, that the son might have come in the enraged pursuit of a miscreant parent. Whatever the man's motivation, he had no sooner secured refuge at the leprosarium than the arrival and murder of his son resulted in his arrest and imprisonment.

"However fine you grind the inevitable," wrote the poet Taro Kitamura (1922–1992), "you get not a single grain of happenstance ("No. 7," *Minato no hito* [Harbor people]). We can only speculate as to the father's culpability in the death of his son. Let us be careful, though, not to attribute all his woes to his leprosy. And let us be doubly careful not to attribute his fate or, for that matter, our fate, to the doings of others or to cosmic machinations.

The man's fate and the inevitability of that fate were the culmination, however unintentional, of his own actions. He would have received little or no treatment for his leprosy during his six-year incarceration. He incurred, meanwhile, the additional curse of tuberculosis and encountered the inescapable prospect of a horrible death. We can be certain, though, that those events brought him to terms with his role in shaping his fate.

Two other headstones bore visages and names that identified their graves' occupants as Korean. Most of the headstones bore no visages, however, and offered only inconclusive evidence of ethnicity, but we knew that people from the Korean peninsula accounted for at least a significant minority in the cemetery's population.

In 1937, Stalin forcibly moved more than 170,000 ethnic Koreans who lived in the Soviet Far East to Soviet republics in Central Asia. Stalin was pathologically suspicious, and the ostensible reason for the forced migration was fear of infiltration from Japanese-occupied Manchuria and Korea. The event occurred at the height of his purges, and the Soviet dictator cast his net wide, dealing with the suspect East Asians en masse rather than individually.

Countless individuals died during the first year while tackling the seemingly insane task of trying to convert desert into cropland. The ethnic Koreans who survived worked hand in hand with similarly displaced ethnic Chechnyans, Crimeans, Germans, Turks, and others. Together, they built irrigation systems and expanded the reach of arable land. We therefore suspect that Stalin's chief motivation for the forced migration was agriculture, rather than national security.

No repatriation was in store for the ethnic Koreans at the end of World War II. They shared the constraints on mobility experienced by all citizens of the Soviet Union. And their offspring occupy several graves in the Kutschurgan cemetery.

Yohei, as usual, wanted to meet with residents. A smiling nurse proffered a white frock, but he declined, insisting that he preferred to make the rounds in his ordinary attire.

"Why," Yohei asked me once outside, "would they want to dress me in white, even though I'm not a physician?"

Yohei set off at a brisk pace toward the residents' homes. He detested the white garb because he regarded it as a mode of asserting authority over patients and former patients.

Russia and the other former members of the Soviet Union had officially achieved the elimination of leprosy. We wondered, however, if it didn't harbor numerous unreported cases, just as we had discovered that Brazil did.

The MDT had arrived in the 15 former republics of the Soviet Union only through the efforts of the Drabiks. The WHO had been remiss in its duty there. What we had seen called into question the WHO's integrity in handling the funding provided by the Nippon Foundation. Distributing the MDT blister packs sooner would have reduced the incidence of aftereffects. It would have allowed more patients to return unashamedly to society and to their families.

Russia and its vassal states remained basically closed to the world. Yohei was seeking to pry them open. That was the sense of mission that I perceived in his every act and word during our visit.

8

UNFORGETTABLE PEOPLE
KARAKALPAKSTAN (UZBEKISTAN) AND TAJIKISTAN, SPAIN AND PORTUGAL, DEMOCRATIC REPUBLIC OF THE CONGO

"This was a thriving fishing port. Here was a landing for the boats. When I was little, we'd dive into the sea from here."

The "sea" was the Aral. The speaker was one of our escorts in Karakalpakstan. The setting was desert, the exposed bed of what was once a vast lake. The scenery was an appalling array of rusting hulks of fishing boats that the shrinkage of the lake had rendered obsolete. The municipality was Muynak. The date was July 5, 2013. The time of day was just shy of noon.

"Food processing was a big industry in Muynak," continued the escort. "We had a big cannery, and it exported 20 million cans a year of fish in tomato sauce and other fish products. Muynak was a prosperous city. It had a population of around 70,000 until the 1980s, and about 40% of the residents were Russian. The population is now down to about 25,000, and nearly everyone is old."

Karakalpakstan, as noted elsewhere, is an autonomous republic at the northwest end of Uzbekistan. Its northern tip abuts what was once the southern shore of the Aral Sea. The Aral Sea was the world's fourth-largest lake in 1960, with a surface area of 68,000 square kilometers. Irrigation projects diverted water from its feeder rivers, however, and the lake had shriveled to just a tenth of that area at the time of our visit. We had flown to Tashkent, where Yohei had met with the WHO country representative, Dr. Asmus Hammerich, and with the minister of health, Alimov Anvar Valiyevich.

After our brief stop in the Uzbekistan capital, we had flown to Nukus, the capital of Karakalpakstan. Yohei was fulfilling a promise that he had made the previous year at Astrakhan's Institute of Leprosy Training and Research to leprologists from Karakalpakstan and Tajikistan. He had come, as promised, to visit the two remaining leprosaria in their nations.

Accompanying us from Tashkent was Uzbekistan's foremost leprologist, Dr. Eshboyev Egamberdi Khusanovich. Hosting us in Nukus was Dr. Atajan Khamraev, Karakalpakstan's deputy health minister. Also present was Romana Drabik, who had flown in from Germany to rejoin us for the visits.

Karakalpakstan's leprosarium was in Krantau, 40 kilometers south of Nukus, but another had formerly operated in Muynak, 220 kilometers north of Nukus, and a clinic in that shrinking city continued to serve leprosy recoverees, along with other patients. We therefore made the detour to see the former site of the leprosarium and the clinic.

Fittingly, we traveled to Tashkent from Seoul's Incheon International Airport on a flight operated by the Republic of Korea's Asiana Airlines. We had learned during our visit to Russia and Ukraine the previous year of the heartrending story of Koreans in Central Asia. Stalin forcibly moved some 170,000 Koreans to Uzbekistan and to other then Soviet republics in Central Asia. The displaced also included numerous Chechens, Kalmyks, and Japanese. Soviet forces captured hundreds of thousands of Japanese soldiers at the end of World War II, and the POWs encountered a horrendous fate. The other Western Allies released nearly all of their Japanese prisoners of war by 1946, but the Soviets kept most of their Japanese POWs for years, some until 1950. They put the POWs to work in forced labor camps under horrific conditions. Tens of thousands died.

Our guides explained to us that Muynak had been a destination for a multiethnic cast of forcibly displaced persons. Unsurprisingly, a lot of the unfortunate souls had contracted leprosy. We heard that four or five Japanese POWs held in Uzbekistan had contracted the disease. The clinic in Muynak that tended to former leprosy patients occupied a simple but attractive building—white walls and slate roof. It was new and stood on a site that had until recently lain under the waters of the Aral Sea. The clinic served the 49 recovered leprosy patients who resided in Muynak.

We met eight women at the clinic who were recovered leprosy patients and who regaled us with stories of swimming in the Aral Sea in their youth. Some of them told us that they had worked at the cannery and that their husbands and children had, too.

A young saint

The Krantau leprosarium occupies five hectares of wooded land beside a large river. Its lush setting is a heaven-and-hell contrast with the desiccation that we witnessed in Muynak.

"I'm satisfied with everything about my life here," beamed a 77-year-old female resident. "The medicine, the doctor's appointments, the rent—everything is free. I've got children and grandchildren, and I'm free to go visit them whenever I want. And the nurses take wonderful care of me when I get back. I couldn't ask for more."

"It's the same symbiosis that we saw last year in Russia and Ukraine," observed Yohei. "The caregivers owe their livelihoods to that woman and to the other patients, to leprosy. Everyone here is part of one big family."

The residents at the leprosarium numbered 35 and the staff members 97, including 42 nurses, at the time of our visit. We learned that some of the staff members divide their time between the leprosarium and a clinic in a town between Nukus and Krantau. The clinic serves a broad range of outpatients, including former leprosy patients. Some of the personnel, we heard, are relatives of former leprosy patients.

Yohei's mood, brightened by the Krantau symbiosis, soured when we arrived at the clinic. The name of the town means salt lake in Turkic. And the landscape was every bit as parched as what we had experienced on the Aral seabed in Muynak, the sun every bit as intense.

Physicians and nurses scurried about in the sun-scorched, single-story clinic to keep up with the steady inflow of outpatients. From inside emanated the sound of agitated men's voices. Four or five former leprosy patients had cornered Khamraev. The men were angry at being charged for care even though their medical care was supposed to be free of charge. They had taken their complaint to the minister of health, but he had declined to meet with them. Khamraev explained the difference between what was free and what was billable.

"You seem to think that your history of leprosy entitles you to free care for any and every ailment. But heart problems and problems with other organs are not necessarily aftereffects of leprosy. They are separate issues and therefore billable."

Yohei was ordinarily prone to jump into such exchanges, but he saw that he was unlikely to be of service to anyone in this one and heeled about to withdraw. At that moment, a nurse approached. Her facial features were the striking contrast that we had seen repeatedly in Central Asia: jet-black hair and blue eyes that resided behind thick eyelids under dark eyelashes. She reported a newly discovered case of leprosy and asked if Yohei wished to meet the patient. Yohei jumped, of course, at the offer, and the nurse led us into an examination room. There, we found two young men of about 20 sitting on beds.

We learned from the nurse that the two patients were born and grew up together in the same village and that they both still lived there. The one sitting on the bed to our left had exhibited symptoms of leprosy earlier and had since been commuting to the clinic. Leprosy had also occurred among his parents and grandparents. Yohei had the young man remove his T-shirt and verified the telltale presence of white spots on his torso. Next, Yohei touched the man's chin and cheeks to check for rough patches on the skin.

"Take the medicine as instructed," Yohei assured the patient. "You'll be rid of the leprosy bacteria in 6 to 12 months."

The visible symptoms and the diagnosis had surely been a trying experience for the young man, but he seemed calm and comfortable with the prognosis. His companion, seated on the bed to the right, on the other hand stared blankly into space through oddly dilated pupils. At the urging of the nurse, this patient also removed his T-shirt. Visible on the youthful chest were pale white spots.

"Please have a look," the nurse requested Yohei.

It was the latest of countless times that Yohei, though not a physician, had been asked to examine a patient. He complied, caressing the white spots and monitoring the patient's response, touching the chin, lifting the hands.

"You've got nothing to worry about," Yohei reassured the young man. "You're lucky that you came here when you did. The problem is in the earliest stages. Take the medicine, and you'll get over it completely."

The patient shifted his gaze slightly toward Yohei's face but didn't utter a word. He remained silent even when the nurse crouched down and pulled his right foot out of his sandal for Yohei to see.

"Look at this," said the nurse as she unpeeled gauze from the foot.

Yohei took the patient's foot in hand and, lowering his head almost to the floor, scrutinized it closely.

"Ah, well that's nasty."

The foot had a bright-red rupture a centimeter wide in the sole, just below the base of the big toe. Yohei touched the skin around the rupture, and the patient evinced no sensation.

"We need to get this sterilized. But you'll be fine. You're going to get well."

Yohei then rose, seated himself on the bed, and wrapped his arm around the patient's shoulders.

"This young man," offered the nurse in a worried tone, "has learned about his illness, and that has been a tremendous shock for him."

"So you know about leprosy, right?" Yohei asked of the patient. "Has anyone else in your family had the disease?"

"My grandfather," replied the patient in a voice barely more than a whisper.

"You knew about your grandfather, and you thought that you might have the disease, too, so you came here, right?"

"Yes."

"Did other people in your village have leprosy?"

"Yes."

"So you knew about the disease."

"Yes."

The young man was somehow saintly, his dazed look of disorientation a timeless apotheosis of the human response to leprosy.

"You're going to be fine," Yohei reassured the patient once more in a convincing voice.

"I keep recalling a 12-year-old girl in the Timor-Leste district of Oecusse who had contracted leprosy," Yohei mentioned to me as we left the room. "Her case was painful for me to see. If only she had received an examination sooner, the aftereffects would have been minor. That's not to say that she had a severe case. Her only prominent deformity was a small crook in the ring finger on her right hand. But she was only 12 years old. And now I see that the disease is afflicting young people here, too. That's just another reminder of how much work remains for me to do."

Time did not allow for us to visit the two patients' hometown. Yohei had an appointment later that day to meet with Karakalpak health officials, and we needed to catch a flight that night to Tashkent. Otherwise, Yohei would have asked the young men to show us their village. And he was clearly frustrated at having to leave them with no more than a few words of encouragement.

The clinic staff had presumably summoned the two young men to be there for Yohei's visit. Yet nothing that Yohei said was sufficient to restore a smile to the face of the newly diagnosed patient. Leprosy, unlike the black-and-white issues of health and survival that arise in cancer and tuberculosis, is an existential affliction. It confronts the afflicted with challenges to their sense of worth. Leprosy has been a subject of discrimination by the world's faiths, including local folk religions and global religious organizations alike, since time immemorial. That has caused sufferers to question their validity as members of society and their standing in the natural order.

Leprosy is curable. The shock of the diagnosis, however, is an enduring trauma. Sitting on the bed, the newly diagnosed patient was standing in the vanguard of humanity's struggle for validity. I wished him well in my heart as we nodded farewell on the way out.

A compelling Tajik query

We flew from Nukus back to Tashkent and from there to Istanbul. Yohei took advantage of our 12-hour layover there to visit a former leprosarium. After a late-night departure, we arrived in the capital of Tajikistan, Dushanbe, at 4 a.m. On hand to meet Yohei despite the predawn hour was Dr. Azizullo Kosimov, the head of Tajikistan's Republican Center of Venereal and Skin Diseases. We had met him the previous year in Astrakhan, and Yohei was fulfilling a promise, as noted elsewhere, made at that time.

Yohei met later in Dushanbe with Tajikistan's deputy health minister Dr. Sohibnazar Rahmonov. We learned from him that physicians from Astrakhan had conducted a leprosy survey in Tajikistan in 1991 and that Afghan refugees accounted for a large number of the cases discovered by the survey. Rahmonov added that some of those "cases" resulted from the misdiagnosis of skin problems other than leprosy. The health authorities had committed the misdiagnosed patients to isolation facilities but released them on discovering the error.

Rahmonov's ministry nixed Yohei's plan to visit the town of Khorugh, on the Pamir Plateau near the border with Afghanistan. Yohei wanted to investigate the flow of leprosy into Tajikistan via refugees. He had heard that more than 1,000 Afghan refugees were receiving treatment for leprosy in Tajikistan and that a lot of them were in Khorugh. The officials explained, however, that unrest in the vicinity of that town rendered a visit unacceptably dangerous. We traveled instead to the Honaka leprosarium, Tajikistan's only specialized care facility for the disease.

The Honaka leprosarium occupies 50 hectares in a lovely pastoral setting a 90-minute drive from Dushanbe. It commands a lovely view of mountains across the Kofarnihon River. That river arises in the Gissar Range and flows into the Amu Darya en route to the Aral Sea.

At the time of our visit, the leprosarium housed 15 former patients, cared for by a staff of 26. We heard that the patient population had been as large as 170 in the 1960s. We heard, too, that three Afghan patients had resided at the leprosarium but that they had been moved in recent years to a facility on the Pamir Plateau. Yohei greeted each of the residents in turn. One of them presented a sight that registered powerfully with even the field-hardened Yohei. The resident had open sores on the soles of his feet but appeared sockless and unbandaged in leather shoes. We guessed that the shoes were a show of respect to the visiting Yohei and that, as elsewhere, the facility administrators were striving to put the best possible face on their operations.

A longtime resident told Yohei of three former Japanese soldiers who had once resided at the facility.

"Do you remember their names?"

"Only one, a guy named Sawada."

"What became of them?"

"They got sent back to Japan. That would have been around 1955."

Drabik was a familiar presence at the Honaka leprosarium as at all of the leprosaria that we visited together. She greeted the residents in turn with a smile and a hug and conversed briefly with each.

Astrakhan's Institute of Leprosy Training and Research, Drabik confirmed, functioned as a sort of command tower for leprosy care and as a clearing house for patients in Central Asia. Some of the patients at leprosaria in the region arrived via Astrakhan. That was true of an especially unfortunate man that we met at the Honaka leprosarium. The man, a Tajik, was a former patient but suffered drastic aftereffects. He had lost his nose, and his nostrils faced directly outward. He had propped his crutches up against the chair where he sat. His fingers were stiff and disfigured, his scarred feet jammed into leather shoes.

"These legs kept me in bed for two months," grumbled the man. "Even now, walking is a struggle. I keep falling down."

The man informed us that he had qualified as a science teacher in 1961 after studying hard and earning a university scholarship. His voice trailed off as he lamented the detour that his life had taken after he was diagnosed with leprosy. Drabik crouched down beside him and asked him if anything was causing especially severe pain or hardship.

"I can't stand to look into a mirror," answered the man after a pause. "This might sound silly—and of course you don't know what I used to look like— but I was a decent-looking guy when I was young. And now I've got this face. I didn't drink, didn't go off after school to play soccer. I devoted myself properly to my studies, and this hideous fate is my reward from God. My body keeps deteriorating into something uglier by the day. Why did I have to be born into this life?"

The sentiment expressed by the man was completely understandable in view of his circumstances. His honest and straightforward outpouring was a gripping contrast, however, with the platitudes that we were accustomed to hearing from leprosarium residents. The platitudes, of course, were only natural. People don't ordinarily bare their souls to someone they've just met.

This man had broken the pattern, thanks to Drabik's empathetic encouragement. He was speaking up on behalf of everyone who had suffered disfigurement as an aftereffect of leprosy. I felt that I was hearing directly from the collective heart of disfigured former patients for the first time. And the question that the man posed was compelling: "Why?" It was a query that haunts me to this day.

The Portugal-born atrocity of parent-child separation

The Nippon Foundation sponsored five symposiums from February 2012 to June 2015 to help disseminate the UN Principles and Guidelines for the Elimination of Discrimination against Persons Affected by Leprosy and Their Family Members. It held each confab under the banner of "leprosy and human rights." The series kicked off in Rio de Janeiro and included subsequent gatherings in New Delhi, Addis Ababa, Rabat, and Geneva.

I accompanied Yohei to Morocco in October 2014 to attend the fourth installment in the symposium series. That gathering convened in Rabat on October 28. Along with covering the event in connection with this book, I gave a talk on the status and importance of recording the story of leprosy in Japan.

Our itinerary included a medical center in Tangier, where Yohei saw leprosy bacilli through a microscope for the first time.

"So this is the villain, eh?" Yohei bellowed. "So this little pipsqueak, this larva-like runt is who's been tormenting humanity for thousands of years."

I peered into the microscope, too. The bacilli did, indeed, look like squirming larvae. We had finally come face-to-face with the enemy, and it was more pathetic than intimidating in its appearance.

Our next stop was across the Mediterranean, the Sanatorium of San Francisco de Borja. That leprosarium, better known as Fontilles, occupies a scenic, mountainous setting about 80 kilometers south of Valencia. Opened in 1909, it still housed several dozen elderly former patients at the time of our visit and served more than 200 outpatients. The leprosarium complex comprises stone buildings, some built in the 17th century, and has the look of an old castle. Running along a ridge above the complex was a daunting stone wall. The wall looked all the more daunting when we heard a chilling facet of its history from the leprosarium director. In the facility's early days, guards stationed atop the wall sometimes shot patients who were trying to escape, he said.

We headed from Valencia to Portugal, where we visited a leprosy-care facility near the medieval capital of Coimbra. The facility began operation in 1947 as Portugal's only leprosarium but has operated since the 1990s as a general hospital. Now known as the Rovisco Pais Hospital, it offers special strengths in rehabilitative care for victims of accidents and strokes. Yohei had visited the facility 10 years earlier, and the number of former leprosy patients there had dwindled. Rovisco Pais Hospital housed about 40 recovered leprosy patients at the time of the earlier visit, but only 12 remained, aged 75 to 93, when we visited in autumn 2014.

The sanctuary in the Catholic church on the grounds of the former leprosarium bore witness to a history of discrimination. It had an attic-like chamber for keeping the leprosy-affected worshippers out of sight of the other worshippers. The segregation chamber had separate wings, meanwhile, for men and women. That separation reflected leprosarium policy designed to prevent the birth of children to patients. The men and women resided in separate precincts on leprosarium grounds. Armed guards patrolled the crossings between the precincts, and a period of confinement was the punishment for anyone caught venturing into the precinct of the opposite sex. The libido generally finds a way, however, and occasional procreation occurred despite the draconian policy and enforcement, as we would see.

Yohei had returned to Rovisco Pais Hospital partly to check on the status of record keeping there. He knew that the former leprosarium held a vast trove of case records for patients and recovered patients. Those records were a valuable source of information about the history of leprosy, and Yohei wanted to ensure their safekeeping.

An old wooden building that had been part of the original leprosarium served as the repository for the records. They were in a huge heap and baking in the Iberian sunlight that poured in through the windows.

"You need to put these in order and digitize their content," Yohei urged the hospital official who was showing us around. "They'll be a valuable source of information for future generations."

Our guide led us next to an abandoned wooden building. It spoke eerily of how the leprosy policy that we had witnessed in Brazil had originated in Portugal.

"This is where parents [held in the leprosarium] met with their children," Yohei explained.

Amorous male and female residents of the leprosarium evaded the celibacy policy well enough to beget 129 children over the years. Procreation earned them recognition as married couples, but the authorities separated the children from the parents at birth.

Atop a long wooden counter stood a double-paned window. A pattern of small holes in the glass facilitated conversation. The counter was toward the side of a broad room. Arrayed along the walls on the spacious side of the counter were twin tiers of platforms. Littering the floor was assorted junk that had been tossed into the room over the years. I immediately recalled the tearing apart of mothers and children that we had learned about in Brazil.

"This is exactly what we saw in Brazil," I blurted out. "They tore the mothers and children apart, and the children who didn't even have leprosy got thrown into places like this at the leprosaria."

"So that's what this is all about," agreed Yohei. "Policy that originated here in Portugal got transferred verbatim to Brazil."

"And those platforms were beds for the children," I continued. "The children lived here, and when they were old enough to work they got sent out to do menial jobs."

"The only people working here now," mused Yohei, "are hospital employees, and they wouldn't know much about the place's history. This is an important piece of heritage."

Yohei turned to the hospital official and said emphatically, "This is a tremendously important building. Please get it into good shape and preserve it carefully."

The Portuguese established their first permanent New World colony in Brazil in the 16th century and basically had their murderous way with things there until Brazilian independence in 1822. Exploiting the labor of slaves imported from West Africa, the Portuguese initially secured modest revenue from Brazilian sugarcane plantations. The colony became far more lucrative with the subsequent discovery and mining of gold and, later, diamonds.

Portugal left a lasting imprint on Brazil through exploitation, and it also left an indelible imprint on leprosy policy in the South American nation. Yohei discussed the origins of Portuguese and, thus, Brazilian leprosy policy with Dr. José Tereso, the president of Portugal's Central Regional Health Administration, and with Dr. Vitor Matos, a leprologist at the University of Coimbra.

Matos explained that the policy of gender segregation and enforced celibacy reflected a fundamental medical misunderstanding: that persons afflicted with leprosy would give birth to children infected with the disease. "The leprosarium administrators," he told us, "found foster homes for the children born there."

I recalled a dusty sewing machine that we had seen alongside the bunkbeds. It was, I realized with a start, for vocational training, just like what we had seen in Brazil. The Brazilians, at least, had undertaken a campaign to reunite children and parents torn apart by leprosy policy. We could only pray that a similar campaign would arise in Portugal.

What remained of the leprosarium at Rovisco Pais Hospital was the nation's last leprosy care facility. That role would end soon with the passing of the facility's elderly residents. Tereso spoke of interest in preserving the facility as a museum. We agreed heartily with the value of preserving a window on the sad history of leprosy policy in Portugal, but we hoped, too, that Tereso and his compatriots would recognize and confront the continuing implications of that policy for numerous living Portuguese.

A health minister prepared to journey into the jungle

We flew in April 2015 to the Democratic Republic of the Congo. Rain is always part of the forecast in the rainforest climate of that nation. Cloudless skies are a rarity. Rain falls. It lifts. It falls again. So inured are the citizens to the sudden downpours and to the persistent drizzles that few of them bother with umbrellas. They are utterly accepting of the precipitation, whether walking down the street or haggling in the marketplace.

Our plan was to visit a pygmy village. Joining us for the trek were the nation's then health minister, Dr. Felix Kabange Numbi Mukwampa, and the national coordinator of the leprosy control program, Dr. Jean Norbert L. Mputu. We flew from the capital, Kinshasa, to the city of Mbandaka, upstream on the Congo River. From there, we planned to head overland for about six hours to our destination. No one from the WHO regional office for Africa or from the Democratic Republic of the Congo's health ministry had visited the village in an official capacity. Yohei wanted to determine whether the village was receiving the multidrug therapy (MDT) blister packs for treating leprosy.

Rain started pouring down as we left the hotel at 6 a.m., and it became increasingly insistent. Our road was unpaved red earth, and it became a vermilion river in the torrential rain. The route carried us directly into the jungle and ran straight alongside a tributary of the Congo River. Our vehicles bounced about violently as mud sucked at the tires and as dramatic bumps articulated the course.

Lightning rent the sky. The thunder was so deafening that I placed my head between my knees to muffle the sound. We feared for a moment that some of the cacophony was exploding artillery shells fired by antigovernment forces. But it was pure thunder. We saw a stroke of lightning dance around the vehicle just ahead of the Land Cruiser carrying Yohei, Kabange, Mputu, and me.

Fissures appeared in the road ahead, passable only over boards and logs laid for the purpose. Our drivers needed to keep the wheels of their vehicles carefully positioned on the wood beneath to edge across the fissures. The lumber had washed out of place at some of the makeshift bridges, and we had to wait at each for the soldiers accompanying us to pull the wood back into place.

We had passed a few hamlets and calculated that we were about two hours from the pygmy village when Kabange delivered disappointing news to Yohei.

"We're running behind schedule and won't have time to get back at this rate. We need to abandon our plan of visiting the pygmies."

"I'm happy to sleep in the car," protested Yohei.

"That won't do. We don't have food for dinner, and the bridges are too dangerous to cross in the dark. Some of them might even have washed away."

Yohei was visibly dissatisfied, and Kabange offered consolation.

"A little further ahead is a village. It has a health center that provides care for former leprosy patients from pygmy communities in the region. Let's have a look."

We soon reached the village. Yohei bolted out of our Land Cruiser as soon as it stopped and trotted through the drenching rain 25 meters or so to the health center. The entrance was dark beneath the eaves under the sunless sky, and the health center was…closed! We couldn't get in. Awaiting us beside the center, though, were two pygmies—former leprosy patients.

The pygmies, both male, were of the Batwa people. One of them, who looked to be around 65 years old, said he had walked about 45 kilometers to reach the health center. The other, who looked to be around 20, said he had walked 21 kilometers.

Yohei examined the two by feeling their hands and chins and found some minor disfigurement in the fingers. He encouraged Kabange to also touch the men, a measure for emphasizing that the disease was not readily contagious, and the health minister complied.

"Does the medicine arrive here reliably?" Yohei asked the diminutive men.

"Yes," they replied.

"Do you have some with you?"

"Here," said the men, producing MDT blister packs in their hands.

That was pretty much the extent of the conversation. We could barely see down to the pygmies' feet in the fading light. The rain was beating down harder than ever. Yohei grasped each man around the shoulders as a goodbye greeting and headed reluctantly back to the Land Cruiser.

"We didn't reach the village," sighed Yohei, "but we saw that the medicine is getting to remote places like this. It gets distributed for free, so it's available even to people like those pygmies."

"To be sure, we have attained the 'elimination' target," Mputu had told Yohei in Kinshasa. "But undiscovered cases could be lurking in the depths of the jungle and even in our cities. Finding such cases might mean losing our status as a nation that has brought the disease under control, but we've got to keep looking nonetheless. Real progress in eradicating the disease is more important than simply attaining numerical targets."

The "elimination" target cited by Mputu was the WHO benchmark of less than 1 active case per 10,000 population. Health officials in the Democratic Republic of the Congo recorded 3,744 new cases of leprosy in 2013. Mputu reported that the prevalence rate exceeded 5 active cases per 10,000 population in 8 of the nation's provinces and that the health ministry was devoting high priority to stepped up control measures in those provinces. He conceded, meanwhile, that up-to-date data was unavailable for some of the nation's 26 provinces.

"We are aiming for a 50% increase in the number of new cases detected in the year ahead," Mputu said. "Of course, we want to keep the overall prevalence of active cases below the elimination benchmark, and we want to get the prevalence rate down to the benchmark level where it is above that level. But true eradication means finding and treating all the cases that are really out there."

The commitment displayed by the health minister and by the national coordinator of the leprosy control program in the Democratic Republic of the Congo was genuinely moving. Here were senior government and UN officials who were prepared to journey with us into the jungle. In no other nation had we encountered a health minister prepared to undertake such an ordeal. Equally impressive was the uncompromising integrity that Mputu evinced in regard to eradicating leprosy. I wished we could impart that commitment and integrity to health care regimes in nations where the battle against leprosy is flagging.

9

CRIES AND WHISPERS
BRASÍLIA AND MATO GROSSO

Setting up the itinerary for a return trip to Brazil proved difficult. The government there was unreceptive to a visit by Yohei. We were happy to hear in 2015 the news, announced to great fanfare, that Brazil had brought leprosy under control. Other news from the "sleeping giant," however, was less encouraging.

Reports were seeping out of corruption in the administration of President Dilma Vana Rousseff. Government officials responsible for the leprosy-control effort might have been serious initially about having Yohei observe their progress firsthand, but the untoward political developments had surely dampened their enthusiasm. Brazil, meanwhile, would host the 2016 Summer Olympics in Rio de Janeiro, and that would presumably command any surplus energy for the time being.

Yohei was determined to visit Brazil on the auspicious occasion of that nation's victory over leprosy, adverse circumstances be damned. He ended up making the trip in August 2015, but definite confirmation that Brazil had indeed conquered the disease was not readily forthcoming. The Brazilian government's waffling continued even after he had landed in the capital. Yohei had feared that things were not going as well as the government had intimated, and he soon discovered to his dismay that his hunch was all too correct. Far from improving, the situation on the ground had actually deteriorated over the four years since his last visit (chapter 6).

A hoped-for meeting with Rousseff, who was then contending with massive antigovernment demonstrations, did not materialize. Yohei had brought a letter addressed to the Brazilian president from the WHO's Director-General, Margaret Chan, about the importance of leprosy-control efforts. The idea was to hand the letter to Rousseff in person, but the rebuff obliged Yohei to leave it with the Japanese embassy to deliver.

Our visit coincided with the convening of a two-day leprosy conference in Brasília, cosponsored by the Nippon Foundation, the Novartis Foundation, and Brazil's health ministry. As noted elsewhere, the pharmaceutical company Novartis AG manufactures the drugs used to control leprosy. Its eponymous charitable foundation funds the distribution of the multidrug therapy (MDT) blister packs worldwide. The Nippon Foundation provided that funding from 1995 to 1999, and the Novartis Foundation took over that responsibility in 2000. It pledged to continue funding the distribution of the blister packs at least until 2020.

The leprosy conference took place on August 6 and 7 under the banner "The last mile to leprosy: innovation, integration and collaboration." It brought together experts from the medical community and from the leprosy-affected community.

Yohei attended two gatherings on the morning of August 6 before moving to the leprosy conference. The first was a meeting of Brazil's state health council. He had not received an invitation, but MORHAN's national coordinator, Artur Custodio Moreira de Souza, was a scheduled participant, and Yohei went along at Custodio's last-minute urging. Present at the health council gathering, which took place in a church hall, were national and state government health officials and representatives of indigenous peoples, citizens' movements, religious organizations, and nonprofit groups. Custodio reminded the attendees forcefully that Brazil was a world-class laggard in the fight against leprosy.

"Brazil is the only nation that has yet to attain the [WHO] benchmark for eliminating leprosy as a public health problem. [...] What is just as bad is that new cases of the disease continue to occur in large numbers. We had 32,000 new cases last year. [...] This gathering is an important opportunity for coming to terms about the need for discovering undiagnosed cases and for providing effective treatment."

The state health council gathering concluded before eleven o'clock, and Custodio then escorted Yohei to the health ministry building to a gathering of social activists. Curiously absent were any government representatives. Yohei addressed the gathering after an introduction by Custodio.

"I have made eliminating leprosy from the earth my life work. Today, all but one of the world's nations have attained the WHO benchmark for eliminating leprosy as a public health problem. That nation, sadly, is Brazil. Your nation abounds in human resources and boasts the largest economy in Latin America. You hosted soccer's World Cup last year, and you are preparing to host the Olympics next year. But you have fallen behind the world in tackling the challenge of leprosy.

"Lots of nations have faced bigger difficulties than Brazil does in bringing leprosy under control, but all of them have succeeded in achieving that goal. Brazil, on the other hand, has allowed its leprosy-control effort to stagnate for the past five or six years. The medicine is free. And it is available throughout your nation. But as Artur [Custodio] has noted, the number of new cases remains large. You here today wield great influence in your regions as social activists. Please take an interest in leprosy control and use your influence to advance the control effort."

Yohei had adopted a more strident tone than usual, presumably out of concern for the stagnation in Brazil's leprosy-control effort.

"Leprosy is a curable disease. The medicine is free. If someone has deformities in their feet or hands, if someone has white splotches on their skin, if someone has numbness in their extremities, we have reason to suspect that he or she has leprosy. The medicine will kill the bacteria. The disfigurement will stop. Leprosy infectivity is extremely weak. It does not spread easily. Please grasp these basic facts about the disease. Let me know about suspected leprosy in your regions. I will go anywhere to have a look. Brazil has been marking time in leprosy control over the past five years. My concern about the lack of progress is why I have come all the way from Japan. I am prepared to go so far as to take up residence here if that will help the leprosy-control effort. Please don't make me leave my loving wife and children behind. Thank you."

The audience responded with loud applause. And Yohei's remarks would reverberate beyond that room in the health ministry, as we witnessed later in the day.

A health minister's anger

Yohei was a keynote speaker at the leprosy conference, and we skipped lunch to get there in time for Yohei to deliver his talk. From the conference, we returned to the health ministry. Yohei and the Japanese ambassador had a three o'clock appointment there with the minister, Arthur Chioro.

When our microbus arrived at the ministry, Yohei summoned Custodio and the interpreter. He invited Custodio to join him for the meeting with Chioro and to raise any issues with the minister that he deemed fit.

Awaiting on the fifth floor of the health ministry building was an odd reception. A female secretary appeared in the hallway and escorted Yohei, the Japanese ambassador, and the interpreter to a room. Those of us left in the hallway had wireless earphones to listen to the interpretation. They would have picked up any signal from a nearby room, but we heard nothing for the longest time, so I assumed that the minister had not shown up yet.

The secretary finally reappeared at 3:25 to let us know that the meeting would soon begin. She informed us sternly that neither the local news teams that had come nor the Japanese film crew that was shooting a documentary of Yohei was welcome inside. Then, she turned to Cusdodio.

"Those of you here from MORHAN," the secretary said dismissively, "can also wait outside."

Cusdodio retorted with a word or two in protest, but the secretary was implacable. I embedded myself in the contingent from the Nippon Foundation and followed the secretary down the hall. She opened a door at the end of the hall and led us through the office inside to a meeting room, where Yohei was biding his time. We sat and waited for Chioro, who entered so unobtrusively that he was well inside the room before we noticed. The minister was tall and was wearing glasses that imparted a bookish look. He looked even younger than his 51 years, and I mistook him momentarily for an assistant. The 60-something executive secretary Antonio Nardi, who took a seat next to Chioro, looked more the part of minister.

Yohei had received only 20 minutes with the minister, so he moved quickly to the issues at hand: that Brazil was the only nation that hadn't yet attained the WHO's elimination benchmark for leprosy and that the nation continued to spawn large numbers of new cases. He emphasized the need for heightening understanding of leprosy in the populace at large and described the value of sensitizing and mobilizing the mass media in tackling that goal. Yohei called on Chioro to persist in informing the people that leprosy is a curable disease and that the medicine is free.

This was, of course, the selfsame minister who had just excluded the media from the meeting, and Yohei was perhaps therefore all the more emphatic about the role of the media in bringing leprosy under control. He also cited the proven value of mobilizing opinion leaders in educating the public. And he urged Chioro to persuade members of the National Congress to speak out about leprosy control in their electoral districts.

Chioro listened in silence, his facial expression betraying a sense of irritation. Yohei moved on to another request of the government.

"You in Brazil provide patients with only a single month's supply of medicine at a time. That is an unviable approach in such a vast nation. A lot of patients in remote regions need to commute to health centers in cities to obtain the blister packs. Getting to the health centers costs money and takes time, sometimes as much as three or four days. The difficulty of commuting results in irregular treatment, and the patients' symptoms become worse than necessary. People incur problems like the loss of sight and the disfigurement of hands and feet that are preventable. The global practice is to provide patients with a six month's supply of the medicine at a time. By all means, please do likewise here in Brazil."

Chioro's expression had become waxen, his gaze defiant. Yohei, however, was unyielding.

"Brazil," continued Yohei, "accounts annually for one in seven of the new cases of leprosy worldwide. Your nation is rich in human resources and in economic vitality. You are better equipped to bring leprosy under control than the numerous poor nations that have accomplished that goal. Please raise the priority that you devote to leprosy-control measures."

Chioro seemed on the verge of bolting, but Nardi maintained the decorum, replying to Yohei in a measured tone.

"You have called for raising the priority of the leprosy-control effort, but we already devote high priority to that effort. Let me explain our approach.

"We are committed to bringing leprosy under control this year. Just this month, the education ministry and 2,300 municipalities conducted leprosy examinations of children to identify any cases early. Earlier, we carried out a large-scale campaign in January, so we are tackling the challenge. We are preparing to work with 4,100 municipalities in..."

"Just a second," interrupted Yohei. "I have something else that we need to discuss while the minister is here. Margaret Chan, the director-general of the WHO, is extremely concerned about the status of the leprosy-control effort in Brazil. She is coming to Brazil in November, and I'll be back then, too. I was unable to secure time with President Rousseff this time, but we will be seeing the president in person in November. You have expressed confidence in eliminating leprosy as a public health problem this year. I look forward to hearing good news on my next visit."

Yohei was seeking a reconfirmation of the government's commitment from Chioro. "By this year" meant by the end of December. If Brazil was truly on track to meet that target, things should be shaping up by November. The minister finally broke his silence. Continuing to glare at Yohei, he raised the index finger of his right hand menacingly, leaned forward, and spoke angrily.

"Your materials are out of date. You seem to be saying that we have 32,000 new cases a year, but that is not accurate. The actual number in the past year was 25,738. We distribute the medicine free of charge, and we don't have problems with shortages or with inaccessibility. I want you to know that we assign high priority to controlling leprosy and that I am in charge of the control effort. We are working hard on prevention, diagnosis, and treatment. And we don't treat patients who have abandoned their treatment as former patients. We monitor them for six months. In addition, we continue working to eliminate leprosy-related discrimination.

Yohei had apparently wounded Chioro's pride. The minister shook in anger as he delivered the impassioned rebuttal.

"So you can guarantee that you will attain the elimination benchmark by December, right?"

"That's right. And we have a solid basis for our confidence."

"So I can convey that happy prediction to Margaret Chan, right?"

"Absolutely. You can be absolutely certain that we'll get the prevalence rate down to less than 1 in 10,000 by year-end."

Chioro stood and posed for a commemorative photo with Yohei before a framed portrait of President Rousseff and then exited briskly. Yohei then shook hands with Nardi and, retaining his grip on the executive secretary's hand, led him over to the interpreter.

"Let's work together in tackling this challenge," Yohei proposed. "From now on, can you provide us with up-to-date data?"

"No problem."

"We have friends on the ground in regions where leprosy is spreading. They provide us with reliable data about the status of the disease. The minister has said that you will attain the elimination benchmark this year. Will you really be able to do that?"

"Yes. We'll make the announcement on December 15."

Latent cases by the wayside

Those who had come and had been unable to attend the meeting were still in the hallway. Custodio told Yohei of a parliamentarian he wanted him to meet. We made our way through an underground passageway to a parliamentary members' office building. There Custodio introduced Jorge Vianna, a senator from the state of Acre. Vianna served as a mayor and as the governor of Acre, Brazil's westernmost state, before winning election to the Federal Senate in 2011.

Acre is home to the largest number of active cases of leprosy in the Amazon watershed. Vianna's father was active in measures for assisting persons affected by leprosy, and Jorge inherited his father's commitment to that cause. He took part, for example, in establishing settlements for leprosy sufferers who formerly lived on the river. Jorge's younger brother is a physician, and he participates in identifying undiagnosed cases of leprosy and in providing treatment.

Yohei broke the ice with an apology for the hastily arranged visit. Vianna said with a pleasant laugh that things like that happened when Custodio was around.

"Artur [Custodio] is like a brother to me," Yohei responded.

"Then you and I are brothers, too," parried the senator.

"I have been extremely impressed with what I have heard about your work. And I would like to ask you for some insight."

Yohei then confided his doubts about the likelihood of Brazil's achieving the elimination benchmark by the end of the year. He related the confident assurance that he had just received from Chioro and Nardi. And he noted the inconsistency between their expressed confidence and the lack of evidence of substantive progress. Yohei added that he regarded the Brazilian government's survey methodology and results as suspect.

At issue was the suspected manipulation of statistics to fake the fulfillment of a pledge to the international community. That would undermine Brazil's credibility, Yohei sighed, in the eyes of the world. But both Chioro and Nardi, he opined, were wearing the expressions of men who had something to hide. They had gone so far as to have the secretary instruct Yohei and the Japanese ambassador to refrain from asking difficult questions.

"You're absolutely right," nodded Vianna, "that the Brazilian authorities need to be more forthcoming with data. They should acknowledge honestly that they are struggling to contain the increase in the number of leprosy cases, much less get the disease under control. Finding undiagnosed cases and providing treatment should receive top priority, even if that means accepting a delay in attaining the elimination benchmark. Otherwise, we'll have a lot of suffering that should have been avoidable, and the goal of truly bringing leprosy under control will recede further into the distance. I'll go see the health minister as soon as we're done here and tell him the same thing.

"When Lula was president, I exposed fraud in the government's statistics, and 32 officials in the health ministry got shifted to other positions as a result. That was an improvement. But I can see from what you've told me that the situation is still hideous. The health minister doesn't know anything about leprosy. That's why he can speak of distributing the medicine free of charge. If he knew anything, he'd know that we have the Nippon Foundation and Novartis to thank for the free supplies. He would have said, 'Thank you, Sasakawa-san, for the medicine.'"

An awkward silence ensued, finally broken by Custodio.

"That's exactly right," he murmured with an air of resignation. "Things were better under Lula. I didn't get to meet the health minister again today. They haven't allowed us to meet him a single time. They're trying to lock citizens' groups like ours out of the process of deliberating policy. I don't know why they have to treat us like an enemy. We won't stand a chance of eliminating leprosy from this vast nation unless the health ministry, WHO, and citizens' groups work together. My guess is that the present administration simply isn't interested."

Custodio turned toward me and continued.

"Sasakawa-san is different. He's been a comrade in this struggle for 30 years. Things have improved a lot here, thanks to his efforts. But the quality of the government data has declined under this administration. In 2013, we had 1,900 former patients who suffered from serious aftereffects of their leprosy. The number increased to 2,100 the next year. That means that we had a lot of cases that didn't get discovered until the symptoms had proceeded too far. We're talking about people who could have avoided serious aftereffects. That's tragic.

"As for achieving the elimination target this year, that's inconceivable. I wonder what sort of message the government will manufacture for the December 15 announcement."

A spiteful reprisal

Chioro acted quickly in spiteful retribution. Yohei was to be a guest speaker that evening at a dinner attended by health officers from all of Brazil's states. He was to deliver his remarks in English, and he rehearsed frantically in the VIP room until the last moment. When Yohei finally entered the hall, he saw Nardi, the executive secretary at the health ministry, and smiled and exchanged handshakes. Custodio did likewise. I was watching from across the hall, but I could see that Yohei had suddenly became uncharacteristically irate.

"They've canceled my speech," Yohei fumed when I rushed over to see what had happened. "Let's get out of here. Let's go back to the hotel and eat and have a drink."

"What happened," I asked.

"This is the work of the health minister. The hosts claim that the list of guest speakers has swelled to 10 and that they want me to back out."

I felt bad for Yohei. The talk had meant a lot to him, and he'd been practicing on the plane and at the hotel. Chioro presumably feared that Yohei's talk would include criticism of the health ministry, and he therefore didn't want the health officers from around the nation to hear from the WHO goodwill ambassador. The minister, incredibly, had more up his sleeve.

We received a disturbing message the next night from field researchers who were assisting Yohei. The ministry, they reported, had ordered them not to provide any support to Yohei. We were preparing to travel to the midwestern state of Mato Grosso. Chioro apparently thought that he could sabotage the itinerary. Mato Grosso had multiple so-called silent areas— districts where the official government statistics indicated a prevalence rate of zero.

Yohei knew, of course, that the zero-prevalence indication was ridiculous. His plan was to go to neighboring districts where even the government statistics indicated that leprosy was spreading. He would secure information from the health centers there and infer the status of leprosy in the "silent areas" on the basis of that information. Identifying active cases in the silent areas would cast doubt on the veracity of the government figures. If the number was large, it would expose negligence and even fraud in the government's record keeping. Yohei viewed that as a means of pressuring the government to take the leprosy-control effort more seriously.

MORHAN had been critical of the health ministry's leprosy-control stance under the Rousseff administration. Chioro regarded Yohei as an ally of MORHAN and, thus, as an enemy of the ministry. The minister had ample reason to be hypersensitive about perceptions of the government. Poll results released the day before his meeting with Yohei were a damning verdict on the Rousseff administration. Support for the administration had dwindled to a mere 9%, a historically low level. Chioro might have been sensitive, too, about a video of Yohei that someone had posted on the Internet. The video included comments that could be interpreted as critical of the government.

"Pretty pathetic," Yohei grumbled. "We'd be better off without the health ministry. We'd have a freer hand in finding out what's really going on here. Anyway, let's go to [the Mato Grosso capital of] Cuiabá tomorrow. Something interesting is bound to happen."

Silent areas

Yohei was right that something would happen. His visit occasioned events that were troubling for our hosts. The trouble was temporary, however, and the results were beneficial in the long run.

Cuiabá's time zone is an hour behind Brasília's, so our two-hour flight, which left at 10:19 a.m. on August 8, delivered us to Cuiabá's Marechal

Rondon International Airport before 11:30, local time. As expected, no one from the state government turned out to greet Yohei. Awaiting us at the hotel was a message in the same vein from the governor. Yohei had an appointment to pay a courtesy visit on the governor, but the latter was suddenly unavailable.

We had arrived on a Saturday, which precluded drumming up new appointments on our own, so we essentially had a day off. I went for a swim in the pool on the roof of the hotel and then relaxed in my room. We'd agreed to gather for dinner in the first-floor restaurant at seven o'clock. Yohei was already engrossed in conversation with several individuals when I arrived. I was meeting two of them for the first time. One was Manfred Gobel, a physician with the German Leprosy and Tuberculosis Relief Association. The other was Werley Silva Peres, a Brazilian physician and former head of the municipal health bureau in Cuiabá.

Yohei described his run-in with the health minister in Brasília and requested assistance in lining up visits in Cuiabá to observe the progress or the lack thereof in the leprosy-control effort. We had three days ahead of us in Mato Grosso, and Gobel and Peres were helpful. Our most useful contact in Cuiabá, however, turned out to be a leprosy-control coordinator in the state health bureau.

The Japanese film crew that was shooting a documentary of Yohei's work had traveled to Cuiabá ahead of us and had turned up the coordinator through their research there. The coordinator, Cicero Frasa de Melo, exhibited a refreshing willingness to disregard the health minister's edict about not helping Yohei. A registered nurse, he was responsible for the entire city of Cuiabá and for parts of its periphery. De Melo had single-handedly discovered nearly 300 previously undiagnosed cases of leprosy and steered the individuals to treatment.

Of special interest to Yohei was de Melo's work at a health center on the outskirts of Cuiabá. The center serves areas that have a combined population of about 5,000 people. It is in a village in the Sucuri district, a 20-minute drive from the Cuiabá city center. De Melo had told the film crew that he would be visiting homes and conducting medical examinations in the village the next day and that Yohei and the rest of us were welcome to come.

Our microbus left the hotel the next morning at 7:30. In barely 10 minutes, we were out of the city and traveling on a dusty, unpaved road through increasingly dense tree growth. Several people were waiting outside the health center, a white-plastered house, when we arrived. Among them was de Melo, a short, white-haired man. Dressed in a white frock, he had the look of a medical doctor, though we learned that he was not a physician.

All of us who had come from Japan would develop a profound respect for de Melo. His frock was rumpled, as were his trousers. He had a bad leg and couldn't walk long distances, but he was passionate about his mission of rooting out leprosy in the countryside. And he would travel any distance required in his wreck of a minicar to carry out that mission.

Yohei stepped out of the bus, made his way over to the group, and shook hands with de Melo and with a female nurse. A powerful chemistry took hold immediately between de Melo, 52, and Yohei. They plopped themselves down in pipe chairs in the health center and launched into shop talk. De Melo's summary of his work in the Sucuri district resonated with Yohei's suspicions.

"They call this a silent area. Supposedly, no new cases of leprosy have occurred here in the past two years. I'm here because I couldn't imagine how that could be possible, and I wanted to have a look. Leprosy is on the increase in areas around the village, but the officials insist that no cases are occurring within the village boundaries."

"How have things changed since you came," asked Yohei.

"We organized a team to visit homes and conduct examinations. The team also distributed information to raise awareness of leprosy and to alert people to telltale signs of the disease."

"Were you alone in bringing a sense of urgency about leprosy to this village, or did the municipal officials share your concern?"

"I've been doing this work for 18 years. I've seen a lot of programs come out of Cuiabá city hall over that time. But no one is giving any thought to the outcomes. You find a district where leprosy has turned up in 30 households. You look at the numbers for the district next door, and they indicate no cases. No one at city hall was saying, 'Hey, something's fishy here.'"

"We heard from the health minister that his ministry is devoting high priority to the leprosy-control effort. What sort of guidance have you received recently from the ministry?"

"Mato Grosso has had the highest prevalence rate for leprosy among all of Brazil's provinces for 10 years running. This is a worst-case scenario. As for the state government, it has used a somewhat different approach from that of the national government. It has accompanied measures for treating new cases with an emphasis on identifying other cases in the same households and in the same neighborhoods. Problem is, its success rate has been only about 60%. So we keep getting new cases later than necessary in the cycle of discovery and treatment. Still, we'll see a downturn in 5 or 10 years, even with this approach."

De Melo was engaged, in other words, in finding the 40% of leprosy cases that the government scanning failed to discover. Discovering undiagnosed cases resulted in short-term delays in attaining the elimination benchmark, but curing those individuals would translate into long-term progress in bringing the disease under control. Yohei expressed agreement with de Melo's perspective and then asked another question.

"Have you received instructions from the national government to prepare a list of patients?"

"Yes. Brazil has a national database of patients. Someone at the health ministry figured out that it was not getting updated, and a directive went out from the ministry to all the state health bureaus to update our data."

We knew enough from our experience with Chioro and Nardi to regard this news of the directive with cynicism. For de Melo, it presumably was an order to delete the accurate data that he had gathered.

"When did you receive the directive?"

"Two months ago."

"Do you have MDT blister packs here?"

"Yes, of course."

"Do you provide patients with just a month's worth of MDT at a time?"

"That's right. Patients get a month's worth when they receive their initial diagnosis, and we provide additional medicine while monitoring their cases."

"Would you please show me your stock of MDT blister packs?"

De Melo rose and led Yohei into the health center building and into a room inside.

"Is this all? Is this all the MDT that you have on hand?"

What de Melo had shown Yohei was just enough for a single patient.

"Yes. This is all we need, since we have only a single patient at this center."

"Please get more from the city and increase your stock on hand. As you know, the medicine is free. You lose nothing by having a lot in stock."

"All right. But we've never had a shortage. The municipal health bureau does a good job of managing the inventory."

Yohei changed tack.

"You've got a solid platform here for finding and dealing with cases of leprosy. Why don't you get more people coming in who are concerned that they might have contracted the disease?"

"I guess people just don't know about the center. Anyway, I need to get started with the examinations for the villagers. We've gathered a random sample of people, so I don't know what we'll find. When we're done here, we'll do home visitations."

The examinations

De Melo's examinations began with a 72-year-old woman of smallish build who was suffering from Parkinson's disease. Her family had no history of leprosy. She reported that she got cramps in her calves frequently and that she had recently experienced numbness in her hands. De Melo grasped the woman's wrists and her elbows and asked if she felt any pain. She said that she didn't. De Melo concluded after a brief examination that the woman didn't have any symptoms of leprosy.

Next in line was the daughter of the elderly woman that de Melo had just examined. She was 50 years old and hard of hearing. De Melo touched and then pressed her hands, elbows, arms, and chin. That didn't cause any discomfort. A swollen nerve rose up against the skin when de Melo flexed the woman's right ankle inward.

De Melo flashed a disarming smile at the woman and said, "Let's have a closer look." He produced two small glass vials and poured hot water in one and cold water in the other. De Melo instructed the woman to close her eyes, placed the vial that contained cold water against one of her legs, and asked if it felt cold, hot, or neither. She replied that it felt cold. De Melo then placed the vial that contained hot water against the leg, whereupon she responded that it, too, felt cold. Placing the vials anywhere on her legs yielded the same results.

Next, de Melo pricked the woman's toes in turn with a pin, and she reported pain each time. She felt nothing, however, when he pricked the sole of her right foot with the pin. Nor did she feel anything when he pricked the sole of her left foot or the thumb, middle finger, and little finger on each of her hands.

"Open your eyes," de Melo instructed the woman, "and look at your hand. See? You've got a pin stuck in your finger?"

The woman was startled at the sight.

"Plenty of reason for doubt," mumbled Yohei under his breath.

"Your feel for hot and cold is mixed up, and you've lost some of your sensitivity to pain," de Melo said to the woman. "We'll get you an appointment for a thorough examination."

Up third was a female cousin of the woman that de Melo had just examined. She was huge and said that she worked as a security guard and that she had a maternal uncle who had contracted leprosy. The woman reported that she had experienced cramps in her calves since she started taking medicine for high blood pressure. She had appeared in sandals but said that she rarely wore them because she didn't like the look of her feet and because, anyway, shoes were part of her uniform at work.

De Melo bent the woman's ankles inward, as he had done previously, and nerves popped up under the skin as clear as straws. She didn't feel pain, however, when he pressed firmly on the ankles. De Melo repeated the hot-cold test and the pin pricks, and the woman's response was extremely dull.

"We can't reach any conclusions here today," de Melo said to the woman when he was done. "But you've got a relative who had leprosy. Let's set up an appointment for a thorough examination and check for things like spots on your skin."

Yohei became irritable on seeing de Melo send the woman off without providing her with a provisional batch of MDT. She had evidenced a high probability of having leprosy, and a provisional prescription was in order, by Yohei's thinking. One problem was that, as noted, the health center maintained a stock of MDT only for its single established case. Another problem was that de Melo, not being a physician, could not issue prescriptions. Yohei therefore implored de Melo to summon Peres, the Brazilian physician with whom we had dined the night before. Peres had befriended de Melo when he headed the municipal health bureau in Cuiabá. And he was someone to whom de Melo could turn for assistance when needed.

The fourth person that de Melo examined was a 21-year-old male. He had no family history of leprosy but was concerned about cramping that he was experiencing in his legs. Pressing firmly on his hands and legs occasioned no discomfort, and he was completely unresponsive to the hot-cold test. The young man had a dark spot on his lower right flank, but he said that it was a birthmark.

Peres appeared at that point in the examination. He repeated the hot-cold test and the pin-prick testing. What he saw was enough to convince him that the young man had contracted leprosy. Peres delivered his diagnosis firmly.

"Your leg is swollen on account of swelling around the nerves. Look. The nerves on the inner sides of your ankles are as taught as guitar strings. That's a sign of leprosy, and if you don't get treatment, you'll become a burden on your family. The nerves are starting to atrophy. If you don't get treatment, your legs won't be able to hold you up. Fortunately, you can get the treatment free of charge, and it will cure you completely. You won't have any swelling or numbness in your legs anymore. I'll get you started with a prescription today, and I want you to take the medicine for a year."

The young man was quiet for a while but finally responded in the affirmative. Yohei addressed Peres and de Melo quietly in a tone of relief.

"Thank you. You've just saved a young man."

Peres kept his eyes on the patient and continued talking.

"You need to do more than just take the medicine. Listen to me carefully. We need to find out who your disease came from. Getting you well is just part of what we need to do. We need to set up some dates and times to examine your parents and the other members of your family. Just you taking medicine won't solve the problem."

"OK," answered the patient.

The young man was clearly unhappy about the result.

"Excellent!" Peres said encouragingly and extended a hand.

"Thank you," responded the patient while shaking Peres's hand and smiling for the first time since the examination had begun. "I'm happy that we found the problem early on."

"I was impressed," Yohei praised Peres after the patient left, "at the way you examined the young man thoroughly and at the way you delivered the diagnosis."

"He has the multibacillary form of the disease," observed Peres, "which accounts for about 60% of the cases that we see. That means that he probably came down with the leprosy a long time ago, probably when he was 9 or 10. Fortunately, he's still able to work, and he'll be able to keep working. If he takes the medicine properly, he'll have a full recovery."

Yohei returned to the issue that weighed most heavily on his mind.

"We've just seen examinations of four people. Three of them were a mother and daughter and a cousin. The fourth, the young man who just left, is unrelated to the women but lives in the same area—this so-called silent area. Just four examinations turned up two, maybe three cases of leprosy. And we know full well that those cases are just the tip of the iceberg. But you've got only enough medicine here for one patient. That's inexcusable. You've got to get a proper stock of medicine here."

"This has been a good lesson," acknowledged de Melo. "I guess that we should stop using the term 'silent area' from this day on."

Chioro and his minions at the health ministry were perpetrating a fraud that was undermining the fight against leprosy. De Melo and Peres, however, had grasped the essence of the problem at hand. Conscientious work by them and by others like them was bound to prevail in the end.

A whole family

We followed de Melo as he left the health center and began a round of home visitations. Our first stop was a farm. The earth was dry, but several large ponds dotted the landscape. These, we learned, were for cultivating catfish.

The farmhouse was a large wooden structure highlighted by a broad porch and even broader eaves, which lent shade to the porch below. Tall trees adorned with dust stood in the yard and shielded the house from the sunlight. Several individuals were standing on the porch, including a man of 60-something years whose face showed symptoms of leprosy. He was a patient in de Melo's care and the object of the visit.

De Melo had provided us with the following background. The patient had been living with a younger sister in Rondônia, the Brazilian state on Mato Grosso's northwest border. Leprosy care was not readily available there, so he had come to Mato Grosso to receive treatment. His younger brother was the tenant manager of the farm, and he and his sister had moved in with the brother's family two months earlier.

"He's taking the medicine," explained de Melo, "but he's had a reaction that has aggravated the facial symptoms. His arms are a mess, too. They're covered with sores that have just healed over. We've seen similar reactions to the medicine in several patients recently. That's got me worried."

De Melo grasped and examined the man's arms in turn.

"These won't get any worse" he assured the patient, who stared out at nothing in particular through lifeless eyes. De Melo then turned to Yohei and said that the patient was receiving thalidomide for the skin reaction. Yohei knew that Brazilian physicians dispensed thalidomide extensively to treat erythema nodosum leprosum, a painful skin condition associated with leprosy. He also knew that thalidomide had a host of serious side effects.

"Do you really need to resort to thalidomide?"

"It's the only drug we have that is potent enough to deal with the reactions that we're seeing."

"Symptoms as severe as this make me wonder about other members of the family."

"Exactly. We'll be examining them today."

Sure enough, the patient's sister had lost the sensitivity to hot and cold in both legs. She was also utterly insensitive to pin pricks, even deep ones, on the big toe of each foot.

"You live with your brother, right?" de Melo asked the sister.

"That's right."

"These two live together, and the brother is receiving treatment for leprosy, but the sister isn't."

"We've been living together for three years," explained the sister. "My older brother lived at home with our family until he was 12, when he left to make a living on his own. He'd been living alone until he came down with leprosy a few years ago. I was worried when I heard of his disease and began visiting him frequently. I ended up moving in so that I could care for him better."

Yohei asked the sister about leprosy among other relatives.

"We had an uncle and a niece who had leprosy. They're both gone now."

De Melo delivered his diagnosis.

"Three nerves in your leg are swollen, and you've lost a lot of the feeling in both legs. That's a pretty sure sign that you have leprosy."

A breeze caressed the surfaces of the catfish ponds and stirred a rustling of leaves overhead. Sunlight filtered by the trees danced on the porch. Tears appeared in the woman's eyes as she received her diagnosis.

"You can be happy that we found your leprosy in the early stages," de Melo continued. "You'll get over it completely, and you won't have any aftereffects."

De Melo next examined the younger brother, who gave his age as 55 and said that he still enjoyed playing pickup games of soccer. The man had a big scar on his right ankle, the result of a burn from a motorcycle muffler, and was aware of some atrophy in the nerves in his legs. He experienced no sensation of heat when de Melo placed the hot-water vial against his legs at different spots. De Melo concluded that the man was a possible case of leprosy and scheduled a follow-up examination.

Yohei had heard that the man had a 20-year-old daughter and suggested that de Melo should examine her, too. De Melo agreed and had the man summon his daughter. She appeared while de Melo was explaining his tentative diagnosis to her father. The daughter, who was wearing shorts and a tank top, looked apprehensive. She complied readily, though, when de Melo instructed her to place her left leg on his knee, and she volunteered that she experienced frequent cramping in the upper part of that leg.

"Do you know why we asked you to come?" de Melo asked.

"Leprosy, right?"

The daughter furnished a curious insight about the hair on her legs. She said that the hair had bothered her because it was thick and dark and that she had therefore had it removed. The daughter had been surprised when the hair that finally grew back was no longer black but blonde. She was even more surprised at something that she noticed just as she was relating this story: the hair had disappeared from her legs completely.

De Melo had the daughter close her eyes and began the examination. Her sensitivity to the hot-cold test declined toward the lower ends of her legs. Similarly, she was sensitive to the pin pricks on her thighs but ceased to notice them toward the lower ends of her calves.

The daughter raised her tank top a little on de Melo's instructions to reveal her lower back. Immediately visible on the skin was a white blotch. Pricking the skin of the blotch with a pin elicited an "Ouch!"

The results of the hot-cold test, however, were ambiguous.

The daughter responded to the stimuli, but she couldn't distinguish hot from cold reliably. De Melo asked to do the test again. The results reinforced his suspicions. When he was done, he gave his diagnosis to the daughter.

"I believe that you have leprosy. The white spot on your back is a sign of the disease. Your father and aunt are about to begin receiving treatment, and you ought to receive treatment, too, even if my diagnosis is wrong."

"But I can only come here on weekends."

"That's no problem. All you need to do is make sure that you take the medicine. Are you married?"

"No. I live with my younger sister."

"I see. Let's discuss the details of your treatment later."

Even the battle-hardened Yohei was astounded at finding four cases of leprosy in a single household. He turned to the daughter, whose eyes were filling with tears.

"The most important thing is to make sure that you take the medicine properly. You'll be taking the medicine for a long time, but I want you to be sure to take it without fail."

Yohei then asked the young woman about her understanding of leprosy.

"Do you know anything about leprosy?"

"Yes, I've heard about the disease."

"What have you heard?"

"That if you don't get treatment your condition becomes horrible and you die. I've heard that it's a scary disease. And I'm getting scared."

"You have nothing to be scared about," interjected de Melo. "You'll get well as long as you take the medicine properly."

Yohei turned to me momentarily to share a quiet observation.

"I've never seen anything like this household. The whole family…"

Yohei then turned back to the daughter and sought her impressions.

"How do you feel about having learned that you have leprosy?"

"Mr. de Melo provided a good explanation, and I can see that I'll get well if I take the medicine. That's good to know. I have another aunt who had leprosy, so I was pretty familiar with the disease. Still, I never imagined that I'd come down with leprosy."

"Another aunt with leprosy?"

"Yes. So this has hit me pretty hard."

Speaking was becoming difficult for the daughter, whose tears had become a flood.

Yohei told the young woman about Custodio at MORHAN.

"Feel free to get in touch with him if you need help with anything."

The daughter simply nodded. She was about to collapse in tears.

We accompanied de Melo next to a nearby village that commanded a view of the Cuiabá skyline. De Melo conducted lengthy examinations in front of a home there of two parents and their three sons. The youngest son, aged 17, had received a diagnosis of leprosy two weeks earlier. On our visit, de Melo discovered compelling signs of leprosy in all four of the other family members.

Beads of sweat formed and dripped off of de Melo's forehead as the examinations and explanations wore on. He had been in the shade when he got started on our arrival, but the afternoon sunlight was now forcing its way through the trees.

"Mr. Sasakawa," moaned de Melo as he finished with the last of the family members, "this village was supposedly a silent area. We really do need to stop using that term immediately. We'd do better to call this a 'crying area.'"

"The diagnoses need to get started with home visitations like what you're doing," Yohei stated emphatically. "When you wait for the people to come in to clinics and hospitals, the leprosy has proceeded too far to prevent aftereffects. People like you, trained nurses, can handle the basic diagnoses. And you can secure the opinions of medical specialists when necessary."

Examining the five family members and providing follow-up explanations had taken three and a half hours. Evening was approaching. We climbed into our vehicles to return to the hotel. Yohei sat with his arms folded, uttering not a word for the longest time. When he finally spoke, he began with an uncharacteristic sigh. It betrayed a momentary sense of awe at the immensity of the task that he had undertaken.

"I guess that I'm just going to have to live to 200."

A ray of light

Back at the hotel, Yohei received a visit from a surprising guest: José Pedro Gonçalves Taques, the governor of Mato Grosso. Taques was wearing a dark-blue polo shirt and was with his wife. He had come at the urging of Peres, who was also present. The governor and Yohei, accompanied by Custodio and by Nippon Foundation Executive Director Tatsuya Tanami, were soon seated in the hotel lobby engaged in heart-to-heart conversation.

191

Taques apologized for having failed to greet Yohei on our arrival. He told Yohei that he had taken part in shaping leprosy-control policy when he was a member of the national congress. Mato Grosso, Taques acknowledged, had the largest number of active leprosy cases in Brazil, and the governor expressed a sense of shame about the high prevalence rate in his state.

"What I would most like to do is learn from you and put your wisdom to work in eradicating leprosy in this state. I came here today, a Sunday, to convey to you that message."

The governor was clearly sincere, and his wife appeared to share his sense of urgency about addressing the problem. Yohei responded to the positive input with a firm rejoinder.

"Achieving a dramatic reduction in leprosy depends entirely on the commitment of government leaders. Those of us here on the ground can't accomplish anything if the task is a low priority for the government. As you know, medicine that cures leprosy reliably is available to patients free of charge. That was the big challenge in overcoming leprosy: an effective cure and easy access to the cure. We have resolved that challenge. The remaining challenge is that of finding people who have contracted the disease and steering them to treatment before their symptoms worsen.

"Today, we accompanied a nurse as he examined people at a health center and at their homes. The basic procedure is pretty simple. And home visitations are an effective way of identifying cases before the symptoms become unnecessarily severe and aftereffects become unavoidable. The visitations are the work of the state governments, and we can't provide money directly to state government agencies. Our main portal for providing financial support to the leprosy-control effort here is Custodio-san's organization, MORHAN. And our activity is subject to your authorization."

"The channels for funding," Taques replied, "are of secondary interest to us in the state government. Our primary interest lies in eradicating leprosy. The national government officials are a prideful lot. They worry a lot about things like losing face. But that's the least of my concerns. My only concern from this day on is ridding our state of this scourge."

"Governor, your passion is convincing. Let's join hands in making Mato Grosso a success story of eradicating leprosy. Let's create a model for other states in tackling that task."

"Nothing is more important than saving lives."

"We're here until Tuesday, the day after tomorrow. I hope that we can get some sort of policy direction from you to take back to Japan. Please point us to someone in your administration who can make things happen."

"I'd like you to meet the head of our state health bureau. Our sole goal is to ensure that not a single individual suffers unnecessarily. I'm in the position as governor to decide when we get started anew on this initiative. And I've decided that we get started as of this day. Dr. Peres, please act on my behalf in mobilizing resources for a stepped-up control effort."

On that note, Yohei and the governor exchanged a hearty handshake. The two had formalized a joint commitment that would move Heaven and Earth.

De Melo appeared after the governor and his wife left, and Yohei, Peres, and de Melo held a strategy conference. Yohei suggested getting the state government to set up a four- or five-person project team. Peres pledged to raise the proposal with the head of the state health bureau. He reported, meanwhile, that he had conducted examinations in another silent area while we were with de Melo and that he had found five new cases there at a health center and three through home visitations.

Tanami asked Peres to arrange for a meeting between Yohei, Peres, and the health bureau head by the next afternoon or, at the latest, by the morning of the following day.

"OK, will do," Peres agreed. "I'm also eager to confirm his position on this matter."

"We're not in a position at this stage," added Tanami, "to be talking about how to eliminate the disease. The first thing that we need to be doing right now is beating the bushes for every additional case that has gone undiagnosed. A second thing that we need to be doing is cultivating expertise among the people responsible for leprosy control. And a third thing is raising awareness of leprosy in the population at large through information, education, and communication. We need to deploy this threefold approach, and we need to deploy it on a priority basis in the districts where the prevalence rate is highest."

Peres and de Melo nodded heartily at the approach described by Tanami. Their commitment and enthusiasm, along with the positive stance exhibited by the governor, had restored Yohei's spirits.

"And a ray of light shines," Yohei said to me with a smile, "from out of the darkness."

Rebellion in the provinces

Yohei's itinerary for the next day included a visit to the Mato Grosso chapter of the International Association for Integration, Dignity and Economic

Advancement (IDEA). That organization, founded by Yohei's trusted Indian comrade P. K. Gopal and described elsewhere, is an advocacy group for persons affected by leprosy. We attended a chapter meeting held at a church. The chapter had a membership of about 15 former leprosy patients. Sadly, several of them skipped the meeting. We heard that they were sensitive about the visible aftereffects of the disease and didn't want to be seen by the foreign visitors.

That evening, Peres brought a state assemblyman, Leonardo Albuquerque, to our hotel at 7:30. The governor had encouraged Albuquerque to take the opportunity to meet Yohei. Peres had been unable to arrange a meeting with the head of the state health bureau, but this assemblyman, he said, exercised strong influence over health care policy. Accompanying them were two press officers for the state assembly—evidence that the assemblyman, the governor, or both had decided to publicize Yohei's visit.

"I am also a physician," explained Albuquerque, "and I worked for five years after finishing medical school as a volunteer in the leprosy-control effort. You honor us with your presence here, and I hope that you do whatever you deem proper and possible to promote a stepped-up control effort here in Mato Grosso."

The assemblyman, thick chested, cut an impressive figure in suit and close-cropped hair. We got the strong impression that the governor relied on him heavily for guidance in regard to health care. He emphasized Taques's commitment to tackling leprosy-related issues.

"Our governor notes that people welcome home wounded soldiers as heroes but that they treat victims of leprosy as outcasts. He raises the issue of leprosy at every opportunity in his election campaigning. The governor was appalled to hear that officials in the state bureaucracy had treated you rudely. Please accept our apologies. And please know that we elected officials are serious about disclosing accurate information about leprosy here."

"Brazil's health minister," Yohei recounted, "has promised me that this nation will attain the under-control benchmark this year. That is a formal pledge by the Brazilian government. I hold that pledge in high regard. On the other hand, I have visited 120 nations in connection with my work in promoting leprosy control. A lot of those nations, like Brazil, have large populations of leprosy sufferers. But nowhere else have I seen such a lack of good-faith commitment by the national government.

"I'm 76 years old, and I won't be able to continue this work for a whole lot longer. Your governor acknowledged yesterday that Mato Grosso had the largest number of leprosy sufferers in the nation, and he expressed a determination to reduce the incidence of leprosy here. My conversation with him gave me inspiration. I resolved while talking with the governor to do my part to help position Mato Grosso as a showcase of leprosy control.

"Brazilians are a proud people. Your government has therefore eschewed foreign assistance in general. But leprosy is a special case. It is a humanitarian issue. It shouldn't be subject to political considerations. I implore you to accept the valuable assistance that is available from other nations in support of fighting leprosy. Please overcome the resistance posed by those who would reject that assistance. And please don't let them interfere with your good work.

"Together, let's eradicate leprosy in Brazil. We can't do that overnight. But given five years, we can accomplish wonders."

"The number of registered cases will double in the first three years," predicted Peres, "as we step up our detection efforts. But it will then decline sharply as people receive treatment and the pool of contagion shrinks."

"Your projection is right on," seconded Yohei.

"The state assembly will reportedly hold a public hearing on leprosy issues in October," Custodio mentioned. "That would be the second public hearing that you have held on that subject. I've heard that the first hearing was productive."

"Our public hearings," added Albuquerque, "include testimony from representatives of other states."

"We don't have time to spare on fraternizing with other states," Yohei objected. "Our paramount challenge is the people who are suffering from leprosy right now right here in Mato Grosso. Their number is simply unbelievable. Dr. Peres, the governor gave you carte blanche yesterday to mobilize resources. Please get started by drawing up an action plan. We'll then provide you with assistance in carrying out the plan."

"I have an appointment tomorrow with the president of the Federal University of Mato Grosso," responded Peres eagerly. "His daughter is a physician and a leprosy expert. She'll be with her father when we meet, and I'll convey to both of them what you have said."

"Excellent. But please know that I don't regard the number of cases of leprosy as something to be ashamed about. It's only a reason for shame if you ignore the problem and leave it unattended."

"I agree," said Albuquerque. "We need to provide the populace with an accurate understanding of leprosy. And we need to get out and find cases in their early stages. I'll take that as part of my responsibility as an assemblyman. We can't countenance unnecessary suffering among our fellow residents of Mato Grosso."

Albuquerque, Peres, and Yohei exchanged handshakes as they wrapped up their meeting. Yohei introduced Tanami as their contact for future interchange with the Nippon Foundation. Tanami and Albuquerque both asked to attend Peres's meeting the next day with the university president and his daughter, and the upshot was a highly useful exchange of ideas for upgrading the leprosy-control effort in Mato Grosso. Yohei used our last day in Mato Grosso to get a firsthand look at some more health care facilities there.

We learned later that the health bureau had fired the female nurse who had accompanied de Melo throughout our time together. The alleged reason was insubordination. We assumed, of course, that the firing had been the work of obsequious bureaucrats loyal to the health ministry. And we were happy and relieved to learn that it had been reversed promptly, presumably at the hand of the governor, and that the nurse had resumed working with de Melo.

Chioro, in a stroke of poetic justice, received his comeuppance shortly after we left Brazil. Rousseff fired him as part of what her administration characterized as a "cabinet reform." She, in turn, lost power on account of corruption. The senate initiated impeachment proceedings against her in May 2016, which resulted in her suspension from the presidency, and formally removed her from office three months later. Hope of a renewed and concerted commitment to leprosy control at the national level faded in the smoke of continuing political upheaval.

10

APPLAUSE FOR A TEENAGE GIRL
KIRIBATI

We set off for a distant island nation in the South Pacific two months after we got home from Brazil. I barely knew of the nation of Kiribati until I heard from Yohei that we would be going there—just like I had barely known of Burkina Faso or Malawi until this project took me to those African nations. Kiribati, I soon learned, is an archipelago that straddles the equator.

"Whereabouts is the place?" I asked.

"Straight south of Hawaii," replied Yohei. "Right on the equator. It's a bunch of islands that consist of coral reefs."

"So it's down around Tuvalu and Vanuatu, right? Haven't I heard something about it sinking into the ocean?"

"That's right. The capital is on the lower portion of Tarawa Atoll, South Tarawa, and the whole atoll will be almost completely under water by 2050. The government has bought some land in Fiji to move the whole populace there.

"Kiribati. . . ."

"It's a bunch of little islands scattered across a vast expanse. I've heard that getting from the west end to the east end takes a week. As an exclusive economic zone, it's the 12th largest in the world."

I was struggling to come to terms with the geography. We wouldn't be traveling, of course to all of the islands, but simply getting to the capital from Japan would take three days.

"What's happening with leprosy there?" I asked.

"I suspect that the nation has a lot of undiagnosed cases. Kiribati covers an incredible swath, though most of its territory is ocean, and the Ministry of Health and Medical Services has only three people to handle leprosy. They can't possibly cover all the islands from one end of the nation to the other."

Kiribati lies in a region that the WHO serves as the Western Pacific. New cases of leprosy in that region peaked at 6,190 in 2006 and declined to 5,055 in 2010 and to 4,337 in 2014. A WHO report, however, cited the strong possibility of numerous undetected cases in the Western Pacific.

The number of new cases in Kiribati in 2014 was 123. Alarmingly, children accounted for 42 of those cases, a far higher percentage than the global average. Leprosy has an extremely long incubation period: 5 to 15 years from infection to the onset of symptoms. A child who contracted the disease at birth would begin to display symptoms sometime between the ages of 4 and 14.

"We can see easily enough how you could end up with a large percentage of child patients," explained Yohei. "You've got kids living with parents or grandparents who are undetected cases. When the kids get the disease, you happen to notice their symptoms because you've got maybe better screening for schoolchildren than for adults. This will be my first visit to Kiribati. I'm eager to see how a nation of scattered islands copes with leprosy as a public health issue."

A look at Oceania on a map reveals a string of islands that stretches eastward from New Guinea: the Solomon Islands, Tuvalu, Samoa, Tonga, and then the little constellation of atolls that is Kiribati. The nation consists mainly of the islands formerly known as the Gilberts. It spans a genuinely astounding swath. Kiribati extends some 3,870 kilometers west to east and some 2,050 kilometers north to south. The nation nearly equals Australia's west-east breadth of 4,042 kilometers, and its length is substantially greater than Japan's approximately 3,000 kilometers.

In contrast with Kiribati's impressive expanse, the nation's inhabited islands have a total land area of only 811 square kilometers—slightly larger than the city of New York—and support a population of 110,000. The atoll of Tarawa, just one latitudinal degree north of the equator, is, as Yohei noted, Kiribati's capital and is home to half the nation's population.

Yohei would travel to Brisbane via Singapore after monitoring the peacekeeping efforts in Myanmar. The rest of us would fly to Brisbane from Tokyo, and we would continue together from there to Kiribati. We who flew from Tokyo took a Qantas flight that departed Narita at 8:55 p.m. on October 17, 2015. After spending the night in the air, we landed in Brisbane at 7 a.m.

Yohei had preceded us to Brisbane, and we all took a flight for Fiji's Nadi International Airport four hours after we arrived from Tokyo. We spent the night at a hotel in Fiji and boarded a small Fiji Airways aircraft for a three-hour flight to Tarawa's Bonriki International Airport that left at 1:30 p.m. the next day. Only two flights a week are available to Kiribati, which accounts for the three days required to get there from Tokyo or, in Yohei's case, from Yangon.

Tarawa came into view through gaps in the clouds. It had the look of a drawing compass opened to 30 degrees and facing left. The two legs of the compass were land, the upper leg about twice as long as the lower. Each leg was thin and basically straight. Even from the air, the island had the look of exposed coral, the surrounding sea an almost unworldly deep blue. The rising sea is gradually inundating Kiribati, and the highest elevation on Tarawa is just three meters above sea level.

Since commercial passenger aircraft land in Tarawa only twice a week, each arrival is an event and draws a crowd. We boarded a microbus under a cloudy sky to go to our hotel, and I soon realized as we set out that our road was the only one on the narrow island. The ocean was visible on both sides of the road, and our hotel stood by the shore. My small rooms did not have a toilet or shower, but it was clean. I borrowed the shower in Yohei's room, which was a detached cottage. The toilet was a communal affair in a separate building.

Just three officials

The WHO's national leprosy program manager for Kiribati is Erei Rimon, a Ministry of Health and Medical Services official responsible for leprosy. We gathered in the local *maneaba*, a deep-roofed meeting hall that is the center of social life in each Kiribati community, and she provided Yohei with an orientation.

Rimon explained that Kiribati had between 100 and 200 new cases of leprosy each year and that 121 patients were receiving treatment (October 2015). I watched Yohei carefully to see how he reacted to this revelation that leprosy was anything but under control here. The number of patients receiving treatment corresponded to 11 per 10,000 people. And the number of new cases annually was 10 to 20 times higher than WHO's "elimination" threshold of 1 case per 10,000 people.

"What sort of people are most prone to the disease?" asked Yohei.

"As you would expect, poor people."

"Where are the cases most common."

"They inevitably occur most frequently here in South Tarawa."

"What about the other islands?"

199

"Lots of cases are occurring on other islands, too," responded Rimon, her expression darkening. "We just haven't been able to discover and verify them. Here in Kiribati, we have only three health officials, including me, to handle leprosy. The three of us simply cannot get around the islands to monitor things closely. I wish we had more people to help, people who have studied the disease. I wish that the WHO could dispatch a vigorous young physician here. We also need a dermatologist. We need physicians who have the experience to distinguish between skin conditions and leprosy.

"Kiribati is a remote place," continued Rimon, visibly frustrated. "We have two flights a week [to and from Fiji]. Getting to our most distant islands takes a week."

"I can see that you're up against a huge challenge here," replied Yohei. "And I realize that we need to be careful not to dwell on statistics. Rather, you need to get out and find the undiscovered cases. And when you find cases, you need to put the people's minds at ease. You need to inform the people that medicine is available free of charge and assure them that the disease is entirely curable with drug therapy. You and your colleagues have the distinguished mission of helping to ensure a bright future for persons afflicted with leprosy.

"I'm eager to know," added Yohei, "why you have such a large number of young patients."

"That's something you'll find throughout the smaller island nations and territories of Oceania, not just Kiribati. Children account for 20% to 40% of the leprosy cases. We're compiling a database of cases that includes such information as means of discovery, age, and geographical distribution. Whenever we discover a case, we examine all the members of the patient's family."

"That's important," nodded Yohei approvingly.

Japan's wartime misdeeds

Breakfast at our hotel consisted of white bread, peanut butter, and coffee. We took the straight road to our eight-thirty appointment at the foreign ministry. Our bus driver parked unapologetically in a big puddle. We'd heard that strong winds and heavy rain had engulfed the nation two days earlier, and the entrance to the two-story ministry building was still a swamp. Neither the minister nor the vice minister was on hand, and we supposed that our appointment had gotten washed away in the storm. The locals joke self-deprecatingly of "Kiribati time." The laxity was puzzling, though, considering that we had set up the appointment at the ministry's request.

"Leave your anger at the door when you come to Kiribati," laughed Yohei when we were back in our minivan. "They say that's a guiding principle for coping here."

Maxims aside, even Yohei's patience began to wear thin when "Kiribati time" recurred at our next stop. We traveled from the foreign ministry to Nawerewere Hospital, near the airport. There, our ostensible hosts kept us standing outside for 30 minutes.

"I haven't gotten a single bit of work done since coming to this island," grumbled Yohei in the 37°C heat.

A hospital staffer finally emerged and took us to a building that bore a sign that read "Skin Clinic." There, we found an angelic girl who was receiving treatment. We learned that she was 11 years old; that her mother, who was with her, was receiving treatment for leprosy; and that her older sister had also contracted the disease but had been cured. The girl exhibited no suspicious marks on her face or arms. Her mother was worried that the daughter had become infected and had brought her to the hospital for an examination.

"You've got nothing to worry about," Yohei reassured the mother. "This girl will grow up beautifully and become a loving wife."

The next patient was a 16-year-old boy. He displayed telltale marks on his nose and all across his face, which had appeared about a week earlier. The boy had earlier received a diagnosis of leprosy and had therefore withdrawn from school and checked into the hospital for treatment.

Yohei took the boy's hand and asked, "Have you ever had this disease before?"

"No," replied the boy, looking somewhat nervous. He relaxed, however, with reassurance from Yohei.

"These are side effects of the medicine that you've taken. You'll be fine. You've got nothing to worry about."

We also saw another young male, whose age I neglected to ask. He had been receiving treatment for six years for an inflammation on his skin.

The staff showed us a computer display of the database that Rimon had described on the previous day. They had input data for all the cases discovered since 2000, and we were relieved at the trend that the data revealed. The incidence rate for ongoing cases had declined since 2009. Yohei delivered hearty praise to the staff at the clinic.

"I see that you examine all the family members of the patients that come here. That is extremely important. In a lot of nations, the examination goes only as far as the individual patient, and that allows tragedies to occur that could have been prevented. I saw that just two months ago in Brazil. When physicians examined the family members of former patients, they sometimes found that all of them had the disease. We saw this not in just one household but in several. Here in Kiribati, you know that a patient's family members are at risk of having the disease, too. And you are doing valuable work in following up with examinations for all of those potential cases."

We moved from the hospital to the village of Bonriki, right in front of the airport, to meet with a former patient. On the way, we saw piglets and chickens in the cool shade provided by palm trees, papaya trees, and banana plants. Amid the dwellings, which had raised floors and low roofs, was an arbor of sorts where people in the neighborhood came to chat and to nap. Women and children were lolling there in the breeze.

The former patient, a 26-year-old male who looked more like 60, was awaiting Yohei in one of the dwellings. He was sitting with his emaciated legs thrust forward. We heard from the man that he was divorced, and Yohei was relieved to hear that the divorce had occurred before the onset of leprosy. The man's legs were paralyzed, rendering him unable to walk on his own. He looked forward to outings when a friend would push him in a wheelchair. The man lived with his father, and all their relatives lived in the village, too, so he felt secure.

"I received a diagnosis of leprosy in 2011," the man recounted, "but I think that I had gotten the disease four or five years earlier. I had surgery for arthritis in my legs, and the paralysis occurred later."

"I'm not sure that the paralysis was a direct result of the leprosy," Yohei mumbled under his breath. He then addressed the man directly and asked about his medication. The man produced a packet of pills from his pocket. "I always have these with me." The man's father then appeared and related an appalling story in a low voice.

"We hear that the Japanese soldiers did horrible things to sufferers of leprosy during World War II. When they heard that someone had the disease, they would throw that person in a fire. Lots of Kiribatis got burned alive. The leader of the Japanese troops was a man named something like Hanasanatan. When I heard that Japanese were coming to see my son, I was a little scared. I'm glad to see that you've come to take care of his illness."

The father's tale was impossible to corroborate, but the telling and retelling of a story like that suggests a basis in fact. Japan unquestionably asserted a strong presence in Kiribati, and that presence was violent in the extreme. The journalist Manabu Kitaguchi (born 1959) did pioneering research into the Japanese activity on the islands. He published his findings in the September 1996 issue of the monthly magazine *Gekkan Pacifica* in an article titled "*Haisen kara gojuichinen—Minami Taiheiyo, wasurerareta hitobito*" (Fifty-one years after the defeat—the forgotten people of the South Pacific).

Kitaguchi writes that Japan's military occupied Tarawa Atoll and, to the west, Banaba Island shortly after the outbreak of war with the United States. The occupation was bloodless, and Japanese mining interests were already engaged in extracting phosphate ore on Banaba Island. Japan had dispatched a lot of laborers, mainly from Okinawa, to perform the mining work. It forcibly moved the starving native populace of Banaba to Tarawa and to other islands.

When the supply of labor on Banaba became insufficient, Japan shanghaied men from Tarawa and from other nearby islands. The Japanese became concerned when the war ended in August 1945, according to Kitaguchi, about covering up their cruelty. So they slaughtered about 150 Kiribati men who had been pressed into forced labor.

The story of the slaughter has come down to us because of the miraculous escape and survival of an intended victim. In Kitaguchi's account, the Japanese troops pushed the laborers over a seaside cliff at the point of bayonets and onto the rocks below, but a man by the name of Kabunare survived the fall. He sustained serious injuries but survived for four months in a cave on the island and reemerged suddenly in December. Kabunare subsequently described the slaughter in testimony to an international military tribunal convened by the Australian government.

We had heard from the father of the crippled young man about similarly cruel treatment—immolation—of sufferers of leprosy. Another Kiribati had offered a different but equally appalling version of that cruelty. The Japanese, we heard, shoved the sufferers onto a boat and instructed them to go where they pleased. When the craft had exited the lagoon bounded by the atoll, the Japanese raked it with machine gun fire and killed all those aboard. This latter version would seem to be a variant of the account of the slaughter of the laborers. Whichever account is more authentic, the peaceful and easygoing Kiribatis clearly have ample reason to rue the Japanese history on their islands.

From Bonriki, we accompanied Yohei to meet a former leprosy patient who ran a small business with assistance from the New Zealand–based Pacific Leprosy Foundation. The former patient, a 62-year-old male, worked out of a shed that stood alongside the road beneath tall palm trees. He earned a living washing cars and filling tires with an air compressor.

We bid farewell to the entrepreneur and, after lunch, proceeded to the village of Teaoraereke. There, we visited a gathering place where the Pacific Leprosy Foundation was conducting examinations to screen for leprosy. About 100 residents, mainly female, had gathered and were receiving examinations in turn. Interestingly, the medical group billed its offering as a "skincare camp" rather than as "leprosy examinations."

"That's the wisdom of experience," lauded Yohei. "You might not get anyone to come if you said you were looking for leprosy. That's why they say 'skincare.' Lots of women have come. When you get women, you get their husbands and sons, too. The daughters are the first ones in line. That's impressive."

The examinations on the day we visited turned up one new case, a girl who looked to be in her mid-teens. She had acne-like blemishes on her face. Yohei offered reassurance.

"You're lucky that they found this early."

The girl's worried expression persisted. We who had been with Yohei in Brazil recalled the expression on the 20-year-old woman that we had seen in the Brazilian state of Mato Grosso.

Joy at the bestowal of medication

The experience in Brazil was a weighty memory for Yohei and for the rest of our party in Kiribati. We could see that Kiribati had not brought leprosy under control and that new cases were more than "likely;" that they were inevitable. The resources deployed against leprosy in this island nation were grossly insufficient.

Brazil, problems notwithstanding, had deployed numerous physicians and nurses in its leprosy-control effort. Kiribati, a nation of sometimes barely accessible islands, had deployed only two physicians in its inaptly named leprosy-control program. At this rate, latent cases would become active cases at an escalating pace, and the problem could attain crisis proportions.

We took a boat the next morning across the atoll's lagoon to North Tarawa. The emerald-green water was stunningly beautiful under the clear sky. Several thoughts came to mind as we made the passage.

I had walked down at 5 a.m. to where the waves were breaking on the beach. Several people were strolling leisurely on the sand flats exposed by the low tide. The previous day, I had seen people basking in the seawater at dusk while holding small children to their bosoms. They appeared to be using the sea as a bath and perhaps as a toilet, though I decided not to devote much thought to the latter possibility. Others were catching four or five fish each in small nets for their suppers.

The people were totally in tune with nature. They knew that time was running out for the atoll as above-water terra, but no one seemed to be racing to corner the islands' resources. Everyone seemed satisfied with what was just enough to get by.

We had been interested to see at Nawerewere Hospital and in the village of Bonriki if those affected by leprosy here experienced discrimination. It might still be a problem under the surface, but nearly everyone we asked answered in the negative. "It might have been a problem in the past," we heard, "but not now."

Sharing came naturally to the islanders. The spirit of "What's yours is mine, and what's mine is yours" was pervasive. I sensed that the faint delineation between the self and others figured in the spiritual tranquility and the harmony with nature on view here. The thought occurred that people here might be accepting of leprosy as part of the natural scheme of events.

We were traveling to North Tarawa to visit a health center run by the Pacific Leprosy Foundation on the islet of Abaokoro. Bridges linked the islets of South Tarawa, where the government functions resided, but Abaokoro was accessible only by water.

Our boat proceeded steadily over the water, sometimes seeming to slice through a taut, emerald-green film, sometimes seeming to skim over the surface of the sea. When we were halfway across the lagoon, the boat slowed and came to a stop. The boatman handed Yohei a rolled pandanus leaf, which we learned was a talisman.

"Say a prayer to the spirits of the North Tarawan ancestors," instructed the boatman, "and toss this into the sea. That is to ask the spirits for safe passage across the water."

This was our introduction to North Tarawa's ancestor worship, which was unlike anything in South Tarawa. Travelers assumed the presence of ancestral spirits in the water and paid their respects like this as a matter of course.

Neither harbor nor landing pier nor transfer skiff awaited us in North Tarawa. We climbed out of the boat and waded through water up to our hips and onto the white-sand shore. There, we climbed into the bed of a pickup truck for a three-minute ride on a narrow lane through a palm grove to the health center.

Three female nurses greeted Yohei at a clean, white-walled building. On the wall at the entrance were a poster that cautioned of the dangers of smoking and the center's densely packed schedule for the week.

"You work hard here, don't you?" opened Yohei with a smile. "I bet you wish you had more hours in the day."

The health center served four villages that had a combined population of about 5,000. More than 10 leprosy patients commuted to the center for treatment. Yohei was happy when a nurse opened a cabinet to show him a properly maintained store of multidrug therapy (MDT) blister packs.

Several patients were at the center, and we moved to a small building nearby. There, a woman of about 60 and a boy were reclining on low platforms that served as beds. The woman sat up as Yohei approached. She, like most Kiribatis, was monolingual, so our interpreter, Kimiyo Machida, translated between Japanese and English for Yohei and Rimon, and Rimon translated between English and Kiribati for Machida and the patients.

"Do any of your family members also come here?" Yohei asked the woman.

"No."

"Did you have examinations for screening?"

"Yes."

"Did your family members also have screening examinations?"

"Just me."

The woman was receiving treatment for leprosy. She turned to the boy next to her, who had been watching us with a friendly look.

"This boy," she told us, "is also a patient. He's 6."

Yohei looked over the boy, who was shirtless. The boy had white splotches on both shoulders and also on his upper arms and legs. He had no feeling at those places when touched there, neither pain nor itching. We were appalled anew at the number of young patients here, this one only 6. The boy had been taking medication for three months. He was the only one at his school, we heard, who had contracted leprosy.

"Are you attending school?" asked Yohei.

"Yes, I go to school."

"Do the other kids there tease you or make fun of you?"

"No one makes trouble for me."

The boy peered intently at Yohei through clear eyes under thick eyelids. Rimon cast a worried gaze at the boy. Yohei turned to her and returned to a recurring theme.

"This child says that he hasn't experienced any discrimination. I'm sorry to dwell on this, but are people here in Kiribati really that free of prejudice about leprosy?"

"As said yesterday, discrimination seems to have been a problem here a long time ago," Rimon replied. "But people here have learned the truth about leprosy. I have never heard of any discrimination.

"A bigger concern is why we have so many children with the disease," she continued. "We examine the parents [of child patients], and we frequently find that they don't have the disease and never have. The same for the grandparents. That said, a lot of the young patients have gotten their leprosy from family members. We've got to put an end to this tragedy [however the disease gets passed]."

Back at the health center, a nurse told Yohei of another person she wanted him to meet. The nurse then brought a woman who looked to be in her late-30s from the back of the room.

"What seems to be the matter," Yohei asked the woman gently.

"No, not the mother," corrected the nurse. "We'd like you to have a look at her daughter."

The nurse then took the shoulder of a girl who had been hiding behind the woman and nudged her out before Yohei.

"I came here today," the woman explained, "because I was concerned that I might have contracted leprosy. They examined me and determined that I didn't have the disease. I brought my daughter along because I was concerned about her, too. They examined her and decided that she might have the disease."

We heard that a great-grandmother of the woman had contracted the disease and had been committed to an isolation facility for leprosy patients. That facility was on the Fijian island of Makogai. The woman had heard she could get over leprosy without any aftereffects if it was discovered early, so she had come to the center for an examination. She earned a clean bill of health only to learn to her dismay that her daughter might have the disease. The nurses lacked confidence in their diagnosis and wanted Yohei to have a look at the girl.

"I'm amazed that you've achieved such a high level of leprosy awareness on this remote island," declared Yohei in an impassioned voice to all present. "That's a tribute to excellent work by you nurses and by the Ministry of Health and Medical Services."

Yohei then addressed the woman.

"You can put your heart at ease. You did the right thing in bringing your daughter here. With us today is Dr. Nishikiori, the coordinator from the WHO Regional Office for the Western Pacific. Let's have him look at your daughter."

The physician Nobuyuki Nishikiori had accompanied us throughout our inspection tour of Kiribati. A Japanese of around 40, he worked out of the WHO office in Manilla and had joined us as part of an extended sequence of visitations to Pacific islands. The girl, who was 16 and seemed on the verge of tears, displayed no outward symptoms of leprosy. Nishikiori sat her in a chair and had her close her eyes. He looked carefully at her face and chin and at her entire back, touching several places and asking if she felt any pain. Nishikiori also touched several places on her arms and legs.

"You can open your eyes now," he said to the girl when he was done. "You have two places that don't have any sensation. That suggests that you might have leprosy. I'd guess that you've had those symptoms for about a year."

"You've got nothing to fear," added Yohei, "nothing to worry about. We have medicine to treat the disease, and you can get it free here. Take the medicine, and you'll get well, absolutely."

The woman had her arms around the girl's shoulders. Her expression was more of relief than of shock.

"Give her an MDT blister pack," Nishikiori instructed the nurses.

Nishikiori held the MDT pack that a nurse brought and showed it to the girl.

"Listen carefully. You take one dose a day for six months, starting today. Make sure that you take the medicine every day, and you'll kick this thing totally."

Nishikiori glanced at Yohei and continued.

"Let's have her take the first dose now."

My heartbeat accelerated as I realized that we were about to witness an event of profound gravity. A new patient, a girl just diagnosed with leprosy, was about to take her first dose of medicine, her first step toward full recovery.

"Here you go," smiled Yohei as a nurse handed the girl her first-day's dose.

The girl placed the capsules and tablet in her mouth one after another and, teary eyed, washed them down with water from a PET bottle. Applause erupted spontaneously from everyone around her as she finished.

"Excellent, excellent," effervesced Yohei. "You're on the road to a full recovery."

The girl looked doubtful about why the nurses and all these people from Japan were smiling and clapping. She finally broke into a big, toothy smile, perhaps carried away by the insistent clapping and cheering. And that triggered an increase in the jubilant volume. Only minutes ago, the girl had been on the verge of despair at the alarming diagnosis. Now, she was the happy focus of this uproarious joy. The expression of the 16-year-old was the unaffected smile of a girl at her birthday party. And witnessing this scene was my reward for years of accompanying Yohei around the world to observe leprosy-control efforts.

I knew, of course, that the girl's expression would be less gleeful on some days in the weeks and months ahead. But I also knew that she would receive support and encouragement at the health center that would rekindle her spirits. She could always recall how despair gave way to delight on this day of her diagnosis, how applause and cheering from others arrested her plunge into anguish. She could always recall how the loving support of those around her on this day brought a smile to her face and how that smile kept growing.

11

FRANCIS'S EPIPHANY
THE VATICAN

Yohei, home from Kiribati, tackled an issue that had caused him grievous concern for the past two years: repeated utterances by the pope that were discriminatory and hurtful to individuals affected by leprosy. Pope Francis began invoking leprosy in a crude and insensitive manner soon after becoming the pontiff in March 2013. An early example was a reference to the disease in a June address to members of the Pontifical Ecclesiastical Academy. That academy trains priests to serve in the diplomatic corps of the Holy See, and Francis had referred to leprosy metaphorically in inveighing against obsessing with personal advancement. "Careerism is leprosy! Leprosy! Please, no careerism," he had railed in remarks posted by the *Catholic Herald* on June 6, 2013.

The famously unassuming and plain-spoken Francis is the first pope from the southern hemisphere; the first, of course, from Latin America; the first from a non-European nation since the 8th century; and the first Jesuit pope. He has earned a reputation as a reformer, and his leprosy reference was a rhetorical device for emphasizing his sincere commitment to eradicating the rot in the Vatican. Yohei was alarmed, however, at the choice of words by the leader of the world's billion-plus Catholics. He was alarmed, too, at the lack of leprosy awareness evidenced by the *Catholic Herald* in disseminating the offensive language. Yohei expressed his concern in a letter to Francis dated June 13.

Your Holiness,

Felicitations from Japan. I write to you in my capacity as WHO Goodwill Ambassador for Leprosy Elimination and Japanese Government Goodwill Ambassador for the Human Rights of People Affected by Leprosy.

First, I would like to thank the Vatican for the support it shows to persons affected by leprosy every January on the occasion of World Leprosy Day. I note with appreciation the message Your Holiness delivered this year and also the annual message from the Pontifical Council for Health Pastoral Care to raise awareness of leprosy and the challenges faced by those affected by the disease.

Further, I was most grateful to the president of the Pontifical Council for Health Pastoral Care in 2009 for joining with other faith leaders to endorse my annual Global Appeal to end stigma and discrimination against people affected by leprosy and their families. A copy of the Appeal is enclosed for your information.

As you well know, Your Holiness, leprosy is one of the oldest diseases known to humankind. Down the centuries it has caused untold suffering— physical, emotional and psychological. Despite the fact that the disease is now completely curable, people affected by leprosy in some parts of the world continue to be stigmatized and discriminated against as a result of myths and misconceptions about the disease.

In recent years, a great deal of work has been done to tackle the issue of leprosy-related discrimination. In addition to the Global Appeal, in December 2010 the U.N. General Assembly adopted a resolution approving principles and guidelines on the elimination of discrimination against persons affected by leprosy and their family members. Efforts are now under way to see that these principles and guidelines are fully implemented, but it is not an easy task.

It has come to my attention that in a speech Your Holiness gave to the Pontifical Ecclesiastical Academy recently, you equated "careerism" with leprosy. This is a most unfortunate analogy as it draws on deeply ingrained stereotypes about the disease.

While I am completely certain that it was not your intention in any way to reinforce the stigma against leprosy or to cause anguish to people affected by the disease, I fear this will have been the result. As your words have such reach and influence, I beseech Your Holiness to be sensitive in your choice of language. In South America in particular, where there are many Catholics and still quite a few people affected by leprosy, I believe what you said will have had a big impact.

May I also take this opportunity to humbly request an audience with Your Holiness at a time of your choosing in order to apprise you of the work being done to restore the dignity and human rights of people affected by leprosy?

In conclusion, let me reiterate my appreciation for the important support provided by the Vatican on World Leprosy Day. I look forward to working together with Your Holiness for a world without leprosy and its consequences.

Respectfully yours,
Yohei Sasakawa
Chairman, The Nippon Foundation
WHO Goodwill Ambassador for Leprosy Elimination
Japanese Government Goodwill Ambassador for the Human Rights of People Affected by Leprosy

The letter received a reply dated June 27 from Giovanni Becciu, the deputy head of general affairs in the Vatican's diplomatic arm. Becciu betrayed a stunning failure to grasp the essence of the concern expressed by Yohei. The brief note reported that Becciu had received instructions from Francis to respond to Yohei's letter, that the pope was grateful to Yohei for sharing his concern, and that the pope would be unable to meet with Yohei but that the Catholic Church stood fully with all leprosy patients and former patients and would continue working to eliminate leprosy-related discrimination.

"Curt" was the word for the brush-off from the Vatican. Becciu's letter wreaked of the very bureaucratic rot that Francis had taken to lamenting publicly. The pope took aim at that rot in an interview published on October 1, 2013, in *La Repubblica*, Italy's largest-circulation daily. He offered in that interview the refreshing acknowledgement that some of his predecessors had "been narcissists, flattered and thrilled by their courtiers." Sadly, he drew again on leprosy invective to make his point. "The court," continued Francis, "is the leprosy of the papacy."

Yohei doubted that his missive had even reached the pope, and the crude language repeated in the *La Repubblica* interview reinforced that impression. He dispatched a second letter to the pontiff on October 10, 2013. In that letter, he took issue with Francis's reference to leprosy in the October 1 interview. He informed Francis that all 192 UN members had adopted a resolution in December 2010 that calls for eliminating leprosy-related discrimination, that the resolution included an annex of principles and guidelines for eliminating discrimination, and that the measures detailed in the annex include one that calls for avoiding discriminatory language.

The second letter from Yohei elicited another pro forma response that was even more curt than the first. In a letter dated March 10, 2014, Becciu acknowledged the receipt of Yohei's letter and apologized for the belated response. And he assured Yohei that the pope was grateful for his expression of concern and for his commitment to helping former leprosy patients.

The pope flaunted his rhetorical disregard for the feelings of persons affected by leprosy again in July 2014. In an interview carried in the July 13 issue of *La Repubblica*, Francis condemned the prevalence of pedophilia in the priesthood and offered a frank mea culpa on behalf of the church: "Even we have this leprosy in our house." Francis again employed the metaphor to underline the gravity of a problem, but his phrasing also underlined once more the profundity of his tone-deaf insensitivity.

Yohei was livid. He fired off a third epistle of protest to the pope on July 15. His letter described feelings of extreme shock and disappointment and urged the pontiff to refrain from language certain to cause pain and suffering for leprosy patients and former patients. Yohei accompanied the letter with copies of his first two letters and of the pro forma responses from Becciu. This third letter elicited no response from the Vatican.

I raised the subject anew with Yohei in the afternoon of January 26, 2016. A year and a half had passed since he had sent his third letter to Francis. We were in the event hall on the 11th floor of the Sasakawa Peace Foundation Building, in Tokyo's Toranomon district. Yohei was presiding over the launch ceremony for the 2016 edition of his Global Appeal to End Stigma and Discrimination Against People Affected by Leprosy.

The religious scholar Tetsuo Yamaori and I were engaged in a dialog as part of the ceremony. Our theme was "Leprosy, discrimination and religion—is a new civilization possible?" During our back-and-forth, I spotted Yohei in the audience and asked him to join us on stage.

"Can't we do something," I asked Yohei, "about those offensive outbursts from the pope?"

"We are."

That came as a complete surprise. Unbeknownst to me, Yohei and his team at the Nippon Foundation had been deploying a strategy to address the problem. And they had achieved a promising result.

"Our executive director Tanami [Tatsuya] hand carried a letter from me to the Vatican and held negotiations with counterparts there. The upshot is that the Nippon Foundation and the Holy See will cohost a leprosy symposium. We received a letter of confirmation yesterday from the Vatican."

"Yesterday?!"

"All of a sudden."

"That's great news."

"This has been an obsession for me. And our persistence has finally paid off."

Yohei was aglow with pride in accomplishment.

Tanami had carried Yohei's fourth letter to the Vatican in June 2015. Yohei had adopted a more restrained tone in that letter than in his previous dispatches and framed the message around a bold proposal for a joint undertaking. He proposed that the Holy See and the Nippon Foundation join hands in convening a leprosy symposium. The gathering would take place in Rome and would bring together former leprosy patients, representatives of support organizations, medical care providers, and a multifaith cast of religious leaders. It would provide a venue for coming to terms with the status of leprosy worldwide, for identifying persistent issues in connection with leprosy-related discrimination, and for issuing recommendations for ending discrimination against persons affected by leprosy.

Yohei had pivoted brilliantly. He saw that he was getting nowhere with his approach of protesting offensive language and calling on the pope to refrain from crude metaphors. Shifting tactics, he deployed a stratagem of proactive engagement. He offered a carrot to the Vatican and laid out a framework for initiating a dialog.

Tanami, on the ground in Rome, delivered the decisive stroke in executing Yohei's revised strategy. He had brought with him more than just a letter. Tanami met in Rome with a group of former leprosy patients from Brazil. Among them was a woman by the name of Valdenora da Cruz Rodrigues. Tanami and Rodrigues attended a mass conducted by Francis in St. Peter's Square. As the pope passed, Rodrigues made her case.

"'Leper,' Rodrigues informed the pope, "is derogatory and insulting to us former patients. Please don't use words like that anymore."

Francis stopped in his tracks and made, then and there, a historic pledge.

"I won't use that word anymore. I promise."

The dramatic change of heart on the part of Francis set the stage for the Vatican to accept Yohei's proposal. Confirmation of the acceptance arrived via the letter that Yohei received in January 2016. Tanami flew to Rome again in mid-February, after he was done with his duties in connection with launching the Global Appeal. On hand to talk with him at the Vatican were Zygmunt Zimowski, the then president of the Pontifical Council for the Pastoral Care of Health Care Workers (the Vatican's health ministry, also known as the Pontifical Council for Health Pastoral Care), and the council vice president and two other council officials.

"We are in the midst of the Extraordinary Jubilee of Mercy [December 8, 2015, to November 20, 2016]," observed Zimowski. "This is a time for showing compassion to people around the world who have suffered oppression. It is an ideal time for inviting persons who have been affected by leprosy here for a symposium."

Thus did preparations get under way swiftly for the first symposium ever convened jointly by the Vatican and a Japanese organization. The gathering took place under the aegis of the Pontifical Council for the Pastoral Care of Health Care Workers, the Good Samaritan Foundation, and the Nippon Foundation. Lending cooperation were the Fondation Raoul Follereau, the Sovereign Order of Malta, and the Sasakawa Memorial Health Foundation.

The organizers decided to hold a symposium under the banner "Towards Holistic Care for People with Hansen's Disease, Respectful of Their Dignity." It would comprise a combination of medical seminars and human rights seminars, and it would take place on June 9 and 10, 2016, in the Vatican City. The symposium drew more than 250 participants from 45 nations across Africa, the Americas, Asia, Australasia, and Europe. On hand for the gathering were former patients, representatives of nonprofit organizations, health care professionals, and religious leaders from the Catholic, Buddhist, Hindu, Islamic, and Jewish faiths.

Why the pope erred repeatedly

Francis had made repeated thoughtless utterances that were insulting to persons affected by leprosy, and Yohei had issued repeated calls for him to cease and desist. The stubborn refusal of the pope to curb his tongue contrasted starkly with the concessions that Yohei and his kindred spirits had won elsewhere. Witness the climb down by China's usually incalcitrant authorities as they were preparing to host the 2008 Summer Olympics in Beijing.

The Chinese Olympic Committee had issued a directive that banned the entry of leprosy patients into China during the games. Yohei sent a letter of protest to the head of the committee, copied to China's President Hu Jintao and to the International Olympic Committee. His letter demanded that China rescind the directive. Yohei framed that demand in the context of the history of the fight against leprosy and the progress in eliminating discrimination. The Chinese government received numerous protests and ultimately rescinded the directive before the games opened in June. Revulsion at the ill-considered move continued to reverberate, however, through the leprosy community worldwide.

Yohei won another notable victory in January 2012. Sony Pictures Animation was preparing to release an animated feature that included content offensive to persons affected by leprosy. The problematic content came to light in the trailer, and Yohei immediately sent a letter of protest, which contributed to the deletion of the offensive scene.

Francis's persistently offensive rhetoric was all the more incomprehensible in light of the understanding displayed by the Chinese authorities and the Sony executives. It was especially troubling for Yohei on account of the immense influence wielded by the papacy and on account of the numerous Catholic faithful among the ranks of leprosy patients and former patients. The insensitive language by the head of the church had surely left those Catholics with a pathetic sense of abandonment. This was a pope, incredibly, who took his papal name from a saint who had nursed the residents of leprosaria.

We would have expected the namesake of St. Francis of Assisi to put in an appearance at the historic leprosy symposium. That would have been an opportunity for him to come to terms with the status of the disease and to demonstrate a commitment to ending baseless discrimination. Francis, alas, chose not to avail himself of that opportunity.

Profound doubt remained as to why Francis had invoked leprosy at least three times as a metaphor for things repugnant. He appeared to have swallowed at face value the Bible's metaphorical references to leprosy in connection with moral debasement and divine retribution. The repeated admonishments from Yohei and from others had surely been ample, though, to alert him to the error of his ways.

Francis, as a religious leader, was responsible for acknowledging his misunderstanding, his unfounded prejudice, and his hurtful utterances. He was in a uniquely influential position to help bring an end to millenniums of wrongs and to translate those wrongs into a lesson for future generations. Francis had pledged to stop using the hurtful language, but simply avoiding the words would be meaningless until he exhibited a true change of heart and acted accordingly.

A direct appeal

Yohei took his appeal directly to the pope on the morning of June 8, 2016. He had traveled to Rome for the symposium and turned up in St. Peter's Square at 8 a.m. for a public mass to be delivered by Francis. A typically multinational crowd had crammed the square under a clear sky, but the Roman Curia had arranged a front-row seat for Yohei. The mass got under way at 10 a.m., and the pope appeared in his all-white cassock and cape. After a surprisingly brief ceremony, Francis boarded his white, open-top Mercedes-Benz. The vehicle passed slowly through the tens of thousands in attendance, and the pope bestowed his blessings on the excited, photo-taking faithful.

Francis climbed out of the Mercedes-Benz as it returned to the basilica and made his way on foot through the crowd, greeting the worshippers in turn. Yohei, as the pope neared, held to his chest a photograph that he had prepared for the occasion. The photo was of John Paul II and Yohei in an audience granted by Francis's revered forebear. On the back of the photo was the following message, rendered in Italian: "Please don't use the words 'leprosy' and 'leper' in a discriminatory way. And please convey this message to the world."

Yohei introduced himself through his interpreter as the pope came by.

"I am the World Health Organization's ambassador for leprosy elimination."

Yohei then flipped over the photo to display the text appeal. He read the message aloud in Japanese, concluding with "*Yoroshiku onegaishimasu!*" (I beg you!), and handed the photo to Francis. The pope turned his eyes to the plea written on the back of the photo in his hands. He simply said, "I see. Leprosy," and moved on.

And that was that. Total time elapsed: perhaps 10 seconds. But it was a direct appeal. Others in the frenzied crowd were offering gifts to Francis and accepting his blessings. Yohei, however, had dared to challenge the pope with a direct appeal about a matter of undeniable importance. This was surely an exceedingly uncommon experience for the pontiff.

Fulfillment through forgiveness

The symposium opened on the morning of June 9 with greetings by a series of speakers. Guinea's Cardinal Robert Sarah was especially impressive. He had surely seen numerous cases of leprosy with his own eyes in Guinea, where he was born in 1945. Sarah spoke forcefully and at length, going well over his allotted time. His talk included biblical references to encounters between sufferers of leprosy and Jesus and placed the symposium in marvelous perspective.

"Leprosy attained its greatest spread in Europe at the end of the 14th century," Sarah noted. "Municipalities forced the sufferers to wear white frocks onto which were sewn yellow crosses. They also obliged the sufferers to carry bells and staffs to warn persons in the vicinity of the presence of the disease. This practice was especially widespread in Western Europe, which was the site of some 9,000 facilities for isolating sufferers from society.

"The discrimination had taken hold widely during the time that St. Francis of Assisi lived [1181 or 1182–1226]. Francis experienced an epiphany one day on encountering a sufferer of leprosy while riding a horse. He despised those who carried the disease, but something prompted him to dismount, to give money to the person, and to kiss the hands of the recipient as he did. Francis received a kiss of forgiveness in return, which triggered an awakening. The next day, he gathered a large sum of money, went to a leprosy isolation facility, and donated the money for the care of the residents.

"Francis repented his past and discovered love for the sufferers of leprosy. In his youth, he had steered clear of the villages where victims of leprosy resided. But he went out of his way through the rest of his life to serve such individuals. Francis was thus a model of accepting the body and the words of Christ, and our doing likewise here will be the greatest significance of this symposium."

Yohei delivered the opening address. He concluded with the following remarks.

"We have come together to share ideas about providing comprehensive care for persons affected by leprosy and to reaffirm our shared awareness of the pressing need for eliminating social discrimination against that disease. Those of you here today as former patients are courageous individuals who have taken a stand and asserted your rights forcefully. You are leaders who are blazing trails for your fellow citizens to follow.

"As for the rest of us, let us join hands with those courageous individuals. Let us work together to help reduce the suffering endured by leprosy patients and former patients everywhere. I will conclude my remarks with the words of a friend who overcame leprosy. He suffered from the disease after contracting it as a youth. My friend has spent more than 70 years in a leprosarium. He is now 89 years old and devotes himself to recounting his experience to others. Here is something that my friend always says.

"'I have experienced horrible discrimination, but I want to forgive the people who discriminated against me. Forgiving them makes my life more fulfilling.'

"Hearing that from my friend impresses me anew with the strength that humans are able to summon. Lots of people have taken a stand, mustered impressive courage, faced down discrimination, and effected positive change in their circumstances. My friend is one such person. The voices of patients and former patients who have experienced discrimination and suffering resound loudly. By listening to those voices, we can learn what we need to do."

True to Yohei's words, the most moving remarks during the two-day symposium were former patients' accounts of their personal experiences—

how they were going about their lives, how their fateful encounter with leprosy had shaped their worldview.

A hearse instead of an ambulance

"My mother cried when she heard that I'd been diagnosed with leprosy. She was convinced that this was God's punishment for her, as described in the Bible. My mother regarded my disease as retribution for her sins, and she prayed to God for the longest time, seeking forgiveness. I was causing pain for my family. That was the curse I carried as a 'leper.'"

The speaker was José Ramirez Jr., a former patient from Texas. Ramirez received his diagnosis of leprosy in 1968, when he was a college student, and subsequently spent long years in an isolation facility.

"I sought help from a number of doctors and even turned to a *curandero* folk healer. He took one look at the sores on my body and told me and the family members with me that I had a disease of the Bible. He then instructed us to leave. I ended up headed for the leprosarium in Carville, Louisiana, known as the U.S. Public Health Service Hospital. On the morning of my departure, a nurse gave me an injection of morphine, and a priest came in to administer the last rites.

"In the eyes of my handlers, I was as good as dead. They loaded me into a hearse, not an ambulance, for the 1,200-kilometer ride to Carville, which took 18 hours. The last rites and the hearse on that cold morning were my death certificate. Millions of others before me and since have experienced the same treatment."

The abusive handling that began for Ramirez before he entered the leprosarium continued after he was inside. Ramirez likened the collective abuse of leprosy victims to the Holocaust. The experience that he described, meanwhile, was strikingly similar to that described by his counterparts in other nations.

Happily, Ramirez has overcome adversity and built a rich life. He is working as a licensed clinical social worker, specializing in crisis care, and is married with two children. Ramirez concluded his symposium remarks with an uplifting call to action.

"I am delighted to have this opportunity to talk here today at the Vatican. And I am more aware than ever of the threat posed by ignorance. Mr. Sasakawa is fighting in the vanguard of the struggle to [overcome ignorance and] eliminate the baseless stigma [associated with leprosy]. I also continue to fight in that struggle. I am here at the Vatican [in that spirit] with fellow former patients. We are here from 45 nations. We have this opportunity to take part in the symposium. The day after tomorrow, we will enjoy an audience with the pope. This is a hugely gratifying chain of events. But let us remember that we are here not as patients but as fully recovered individuals."

Ramirez received a round of enthusiastic applause. The mention of biblical illness apparently had come as a surprise for most of Ramirez's listeners. Jean-Marie Mupendawatu, the secretary of the Pontifical Council for the Pastoral Care of Health Care Workers and the chairperson of the symposium had refrained from commenting on other speakers' presentations, but he broke that pattern for the Texan.

"That talk," enthused Mupendawatu, "transcended the matter of leprosy. The speaker referred frankly to leprosy, but in a nondiscriminatory way."

Ramirez was a compelling speaker. He was, unfortunately, one of all too few former patients to address the gathering on the first day. A notable exception was India's P. K. Gopal. He described movingly how he had initially hidden his diagnosis of leprosy while he continued doing research on the disease and how he had joined the fight against leprosy and against associated discrimination.

"India still has laws on the books," reported Gopal, "that discriminate against persons afflicted by leprosy. Our hope in coming here to the Vatican is that Pope Francis would take a stand against that kind of discrimination."

In sad contrast with former patients' personal accounts were the antiseptic presentations by the medical researchers on the program. Most of them evidenced little hands-on experience with patients, and some even plagiarized Yohei's familiar appeal. Those of us familiar with the war in the trenches struggled with the urge to flee the hall as they rambled on.

Notably appalling were the repeated references to "leper" by a speaker during the morning session on the symposium's first day. The speaker's obliviousness to the sensitivities of the participants was breathtaking. A Nippon Foundation staff member raised the issue during a coffee break with Mupendawatu, the chairperson of the symposium. Mupendawatu responded in good faith and called on everyone after the break to refrain from using the term "leper." He reminded the participants of that word's history of discriminatory usage and urged them to display a sensitivity suitable to the occasion.

Francis's repentance

The second day of the symposium began with talks by representatives of different religions—formal and not very interesting. For example, the person who took the stage as a representative of Judaism, an Italian, was a mere layperson and simply read a message from a rabbi. The Islamic representative was no better—an Indian who had next to no experience with leprosy and whose only qualification appeared to be that he had studied in the United Kingdom.

I hoped at the start of each talk that the speaker would touch on the role of religion in discrimination. But each speaker disappointed, each rehashing the same hackneyed platitudes. A glance across the hall revealed that I was not alone in my disappointment. The former patients, especially, looked bored with the talks and offered only the feeblest clapping of hands at the end of each.

Things got more interesting after lunch. Former patients took the lead in the afternoon presentations, which got under way at 1:30. Japan's Masao Ishida described being committed at the age of 10 to the Nagashima Aisei-en leprosarium, in Okayama Prefecture. A murmur rolled through the hall as he said that he had spent the past seven decades at the facility. Ishida described how he and other former patients had fought for the repeal of Japan's Leprosy Prevention Law. That notorious law, finally repealed in 1996, had mandated the forced isolation of patients. Ishida also described his ongoing activity in working to secure a UNESCO World Heritage registration for the 13 leprosaria remaining in Japan.

"I am 80 years old now," said Ishida at the end of his remarks. "I have lived my 80 years hand in hand with leprosy. I didn't have a choice. It was not a life that I chose. But it was not a meaningless life, not by any means. I can remind myself with pride that this has been a life rich in precious experiences."

The hall erupted with applause. I caught up with Ishida later and asked him for his thoughts on the symposium.

"I am a Protestant," Ishida replied. "But I was really happy to meet here with [Catholics, who are] fellow Christians. This was the first time for me to attend an international leprosy conference, and I've enjoyed the opportunity to interact with younger former patients. It's been a reminder that I still have a lot to do."

The chair also invited comments from former patients who were not on the program, and several spoke in turn, passing the microphone from one to the next. Including scheduled and unscheduled speakers, we heard from former patients from Brazil, China, Colombia, India, Indonesia, Japan, the Republic of Korea, and the Philippines. A Chinese man showed a brief video documentary that he had produced. Leprosy had left him with a right eyelid that wouldn't close and with deformed fingers on his left hand, but he had built a business crafting prosthetic arms and legs for former patients. The video portrayed him making the prostheses, peddling them in the village communities of former patients, and lending an ear to his customers' stories. The story of a former patient serving other former patients had an uncommon touch that was touching.

"I've been working for 17 years to eliminate prejudice about leprosy," commented the prosthetics craftsman. "I've seen how discrimination and stigmatization arise from ignorance. I'm the only one like me in China who has a license to produce prosthetic arms and legs."

The speaker was visibly frustrated with the lack of assistance from the Chinese government for leprosy patients and former patients. Even more assertive was a female former patient from Brazil, a core member of that nation's Movement for the Reintegration of Persons Affected by Hansen's disease (MORHAN). She related the heartrending experience of mothers and children torn apart on account of leprosy (chapter 7). Brazil is a heavily Catholic nation, and her remarks registered painfully with the participants from the Vatican. This was the first time that the subject had arisen in public discourse in the capital city of world Catholicism.

"We in Brazil have banned [the discriminatory usage of] such terms as 'leprosy' and 'leper'," the speaker continued. "And we need to demand more [in regard to eliminating discrimination]."

The talks were a reminder that serious obstacles remain for those engaged in treating leprosy as a medical issue and in addressing it as a social issue. Four common themes weaved through the comments by the former patients:

1. The number of active cases of leprosy has declined, but the care on offer for patients and for former patients remains profoundly inadequate.
2. Insufficient access to physicians and nurses is a big factor in the inadequacy of care on offer. Even where physicians and nurses are accessible, they are frequently unqualified to identify and diagnose leprosy. A lot of them blithely assume that leprosy has receded into the past and is no longer a health issue.
3. Cases of leprosy are going undetected, partly because of the shortage of medical professionals qualified to diagnose the disease and partly because of a general lack of awareness. We need to regard each newly detected case as evidence of other cases that have yet to be detected.
4. Laws are still on the books in some nations that discriminate against leprosy patients and former patients.

Yohei clung throughout the two days of the symposium to the hope of meeting with the pope. He was doubtful about the lasting impact of his brief encounter with Francis in St. Peter's Square, and he was eager for an opportunity to deliver his message properly. Yohei had met twice with Pope John Paul II. The first audience, in 1983, was as an escort to his father, Ryoichi. The second, in 2002, was as the WHO Goodwill Ambassador for Leprosy Elimination. We assumed that Francis could muster at least a trace of the good faith exhibited by his illustrious forebear. But we were wrong, and Francis did not deign to meet with Yohei during the symposium.

The symposium participants reached a broad consensus through their two days of discussion and articulated that consensus in a set of conclusions and recommendations. Their conclusions were as follows:

1. Every new case of Hansen's disease is one case too many.
2. Every case of stigma and social exclusion is one case too many.
3. Every law that discriminates against persons affected by Hansen's disease is one law too many.

A detailed commentary accompanied each conclusion, and the full version of the conclusions and commentaries appears in the appendix to this book. The participants' five recommendations, preceded by two introductory points, were as follows:

Two Introductory Points
1. Persons affected by Hansen's disease must be seen as the main actors in the fight against this disease and the discrimination it causes. This involvement is a powerful instrument for the recognition of their equal dignity and rights for social inclusion, and for the breaking of the stigma attached to them. This point applies to all of the recommendations listed below.
2. The use of discriminatory language that reinforces stigma must cease, in particular, use of the term "leper" and its equivalent in other languages. This term is offensive for the reasons stated above and also because it defines a person by his or her illness. Use of the term "leprosy" in a metaphorical sense should be avoided.

Five Recommendations
1. Given their important role in their respective communities of believers, the leaders of all religions—and this is an important and urgent matter— should, in their teachings, writings and speeches, contribute to the elimination of discrimination against persons affected by leprosy by spreading awareness that leprosy is curable and stressing that there is no

reason to discriminate against anyone affected by leprosy or members of their families.

2. States and governments should be encouraged to make great efforts to implement the 'Principles and Guidelines' accompanying the resolution adopted by the General Assembly of the United Nations in 2010 on elimination of discrimination against persons affected by leprosy and their family members. These 'Principles and Guidelines' must be fully implemented, otherwise they will remain just empty proclamations.

3. There should be a modification or abolition of all laws and regulations that discriminate against persons affected by leprosy. Policies relating to family, work, schools, or any other area which directly or indirectly discriminate against persons affected by leprosy must also be changed, recognizing that no one must be discriminated against because of the fact that he or she has, or once had, leprosy.

4. There is a need for further scientific research to develop new medical tools to prevent and treat leprosy and its complications, and to achieve better diagnostic methods.

5. In order to achieve a world free of leprosy and the discrimination it causes, the efforts of all the churches, religious communities, international organizations, governments, major foundations, NGOs, and associations of persons affected by leprosy which have hitherto contributed to the fight against this disease should be unified and joint plans of cooperation should be developed.

Here, in the conclusions and recommendations issued by the symposium participants, was an unprecedented repudiation of papal verbiage. The document was an indelible footnote to the history of the Catholic Church. Yohei had won a historic victory.

The Vatican allocated front-row seats to the symposium participants for the jubilee mass on June 12 in St. Peter's Square. There, they saw and heard the pontiff, standing before a rendering of Jesus bleeding from his right breast, pray for the sick and disabled. Francis went so far as to mention the leprosy symposium and the attendance of former leprosy patients, to extend a grateful welcome to the organizers and participants, and to express heartfelt hope for continuing progress in the fight against the disease.

None of us present at the mass knew whether or how far to regard Francis's remarks as an expression of penitence. We got an interesting insight, however, from the symposium chair, Mupendawatu. He and Yohei shared a car after the mass to a hilltop broadcast studio for a joint interview. Yohei reported afterwards that Mupendawatu had conveyed a Vatican perspective on the symposium that was hugely gratifying.

"This was the first time that we really grasped the tragedy of leprosy," the secretary had confessed. "The pope was praying for the success of the two-day symposium. Let us work now to share the truth of leprosy with our parishes and organizations around the world. We were simply too ignorant of the disease. We were stunned at what we heard from the former patients. To think that we would keep the bodies of patients at our churches for years before releasing them for burial…! I can't help thinking that we could have done better. We really were ignorant."

I surmised that we could assume that Francis shared the sense of repentance expressed by Mupendawatu. More penetrating, however, was the enlightened insight voiced after the mass by Vagavathali Narsappa, the president of India's Association of People Affected by Leprosy (APAL).

"This was a truly historic day," declared Narsappa. "[Contracting] leprosy might have been our divine calling, all for this day."

The repeated discriminatory utterances by the pope, I thought, might have been his calling, might have been to bring this day about. Narsappa and the other victims of leprosy and of discriminatory comments had moved on, however, beyond Francis. They had sublimated their suffering and attained a divinity far loftier than that of the pope. Only the divinely sighted, I mused, could perceive in that horrific experience a divine calling.

APPENDIX 1
BIBLICAL LEPROSY

Victims' suffering and social revulsion figure prominently in the numerous references to leprosy in the Bible. The terms "leprosy," "leper," and "leprous" appear in the Old Testament in Exodus, Leviticus, Numbers, Deuteronomy, 2 Samuel, 2 Kings, and 2 Chronicles and in the New Testament in Matthew, Mark, and Luke.

In most of the biblical references, leprosy is a metaphor for defilement and divine retribution. It is an English rendering of the Hebrew *tzaraat*. Recent scholarship suggests that *tzaraat* can refer to any of a broad range of skin afflictions—including but not limited to what we know as leprosy. Biblical misrepresentation thus set the tone for millennia of misunderstanding of a disease that was always barely infectious and that is now eminently treatable.

The reference to the disease is clear even where the word is absent, as in this passage from the book of Job.

> Why died I not from the womb? why did I not give up the ghost when I came out of the belly? Why did the knees prevent me? or why the breasts that I should suck? For now should I have lain still and been quiet, I should have slept: then had I been at rest... (Job 3:11–13 [King James Version (KJV)])

In the biblical accounts of leprosy, the disease is frequently a punishment administered as the wrath of God. Miriam, for example, earns that punishment when she and Aaron challenge their brother Moses, who is God's appointed servant.

> And the anger of the LORD was kindled against them; and he departed. And the cloud departed from off the tabernacle; and, behold, Miriam became leprous, white as snow: and Aaron looked upon Miriam, and, behold, she was leprous. And Aaron said unto Moses, Alas, my lord, I beseech thee, lay not the sin upon us, wherein we have done foolishly, and wherein we have sinned. Let her not be as one dead, of whom the flesh is half consumed when he cometh out of his mother's womb. And Moses cried unto the LORD, saying,

> Heal her now, O God, I beseech thee. And the LORD said unto Moses, If her father had but spit in her face, should she not be ashamed seven days? let her be shut out from the camp seven days, and after that let her be received in again. (Numbers 12:9–14 [KJV])

Even the highest and mightiest were subject to God's wrath and to the punishment of leprosy, as with the tragic Uzziah. He became the king of Judah at the age of 16 and reigned for 52 years. Uzziah incurred the wrath of God, however, when his pride got the best of him and he dared to enter temple precincts reserved for the priests.

> Then Uzziah was wroth, and had a censer in his hand to burn incense: and while he was wroth with the priests, the leprosy even rose up in his forehead before the priests in the house of the LORD, from beside the incense altar. And Azariah the chief priest, and all the priests, looked upon him, and, behold, he was leprous in his forehead, and they thrust him out from thence; yea, himself hasted also to go out, because the LORD had smitten him. And Uzziah the king was a leper unto the day of his death, and dwelt in a several house, being a leper... (2 Chronicles 26:19–21 [KJV])

Uzziah's punishment persisted beyond—or, rather, into—the tomb. At his death, the people denied him entombment in the burial ground of his predecessors and buried his remains instead at a site nearby. The practice of isolating leprosy's victims thus included evicting the living from the community temporarily, as with Miriam, or permanently, and, as with Uzziah, burying the dead apart from their forebears. That practice established a pattern that would continue, on both counts, down through the centuries.

Isolation also included obliging victims of leprosy to proclaim their affliction, both visibly and audibly:

> And the leper in whom the plague is, his clothes shall be rent, and his head bare, and he shall put a covering upon his upper lip, and shall cry, Unclean, unclean. (Leviticus 13:45 [KJV])

Strict guidelines for dealing with leprosy applied to the unafflicted, as well as to the afflicted. The following passage, also from Leviticus, prescribes detailed procedures for purifying objects and the body after encounters with leprosy defilement.

> And what saddle soever he rideth upon that hath the issue shall be unclean. And whosoever toucheth any thing that was under him shall be unclean until the even: and he that beareth any of those things shall wash his clothes, and

bathe himself in water, and be unclean until the even. And whomsoever he toucheth that hath the issue, and hath not rinsed his hands in water, he shall wash his clothes, and bathe himself in water, and be unclean until the even. And the vessel of earth, that he toucheth which hath the issue, shall be broken: and every vessel of wood shall be rinsed in water. (Leviticus 15:9–12 [KJV])

Aelius Galenus (Galen, 129 CE–around 200 CE), an influential Greek physician in the Roman Empire, studied skin disorders that appear to have included what we know as leprosy. He grouped a broad swath of skin disorders as *lepra* and described the occasional degeneration of *lepra* into elephantiasis, which apparently corresponds to leprosy. Confusingly, Galen writes elsewhere that elephantiasis can abate and turn into *lepra*.

The translators of the earliest Greek version of the Hebrew scriptures rendered the Hebrew *tzaraat* as *lepra*. That is in the Septuagint, a work of the 3rd and 2nd centuries BCE. The translators of the Vulgate, a late 4th-century Latin version of the Bible, also used *lepra* for the Hebrew *tzaraat*. "Leprosy" therefore took hold in subsequent, English versions of the Bible as the translation, via Greek or Latin, of the Hebrew term.

Overly enthusiastic editing resulted in the insertion of *lepra* even where *tzaraat* did not appear in the original. Witness the poetic description at the opening of Isaiah 53 of how Jesus absorbed suffering on our behalf. The Vulgate adds a reference to "leper" where no such reference exists in the Hebrew original, and some English translations retained the errant addition. Here is the passage as rendered in the Douay-Rheims Version (DRV, 1582–1610):

Who hath believed our report? and to whom is the arm of the Lord revealed? And he shall grow up as a tender plant before him, and as a root out of a thirsty ground: there is no beauty in him, nor comeliness: and we have seen him, and there was no sightliness, that we should be desirous of him: Despised, and the most abject of men, a man of sorrows, and acquainted with infirmity: and his look was as it were hidden and despised, whereupon we esteemed him not. Surely he hath borne our infirmities and carried our sorrows: *and we have thought him as it were a leper* [italics added], and as one struck by God and afflicted. But he was wounded for our iniquities, he was bruised for our sins: the chastisement of our peace was upon him, and by his bruises we are healed. (Isaiah 53:1–5 [DRV])

Presumably, the translators have added "leper" to heighten the rhetorical effect. The translators of the King James Version, working around the same time as their Douay-Rheims counterparts (1604–1611), were faithful to the Hebrew original:

Who hath believed our report? and to whom is the arm of the Lord revealed? For he shall grow up before him as a tender plant, and as a root out of a dry ground: he hath no form nor comeliness; and when we shall see him, there is no beauty that we should desire him. He is despised and rejected of men; a man of sorrows, and acquainted with grief: and we hid as it were our faces from him; he was despised, and we esteemed him not. Surely he hath borne our griefs, and carried our sorrows: *yet we did esteem him stricken* [italics added], smitten of God, and afflicted. But he was wounded for our transgressions, he was bruised for our iniquities: the chastisement of our peace was upon him; and with his stripes we are healed. (Isaiah 53:1–5 [KJV])

APPENDIX 2
LEPROSY IN JAPAN

The earliest known appearance in Japanese of the kanji for leprosy, 癩 (*rai*), is in the 7th-century *Hokke gisho* (Annotated commentary on the *Lotus Sutra*). That text's subject, the *Lotus Sutra*, has been a hugely influential Buddhist scripture since its compilation about 2,000 years ago. The kanji for leprosy appears three times in the sutra, each time in the compound 白癩 (*shirahata* or *byakurai*).

Burton Watson renders the compound in question as "white leprosy" in his definitive translation of the *Lotus Sutra*. The precise meaning of the term is subject to debate, but that it refers to a disfiguring disease is clear from the context. Its description is notably graphic in the following passage from the concluding, 28th chapter of the sutra, "The Encouragement of Bodhisattva Universally Worthy." That chapter unfolds as a dialogue between the bodhisattva of the title and the Buddha. Adherents of the *Lotus Sutra* revere Bodhisattva Universally Worthy (Samantabhadra) as a protector of those who study and cherish the sutra.

> If anyone sees a person who accepts and upholds this sutra and tries to expose the faults or evils of that person, whether what he speaks is true or not, he will in his present existence be afflicted with white leprosy. If anyone disparages or laughs at that person, then in existence after existence he will have teeth that are missing or spaced far apart, ugly lips, a flat nose, hands and feet that are gnarled or deformed, and eyes that are squinty. His body will have a foul odor, with evil sores that run pus and blood, and he will suffer from water in the belly, shortness of breath, and other severe and malignant illnesses. Therefore, Universal Worthy, if you see a person who accepts and upholds this sutra, you should rise and greet him from afar, showing him the same respect you would a Buddha.

Thus do we encounter in the Buddhist scriptures the same pejorative usage of "leprosy" that we find in the Bible: a metaphor for severe punishment for disregarding or disrespecting the holy teachings. The renowned etymologist

Shizuka Shirakawa offers an insightful analysis of the leprosy kanji in his analytical kanji dictionary *Jito* (Tokyo: Heibonsha, 1984; in Japanese). According to Shirakawa, the inner component of the kanji, 頼, refers to divine bestowal. The outer component, 疒, is the radical for disease, so the kanji carries the meaning "heavenly imposed disease."

Despite the prejudice against leprosy victims expressed in the Buddhist scriptures, the religion also spawned a spirit of compassion for those afflicted by the disease. Epitomizing that spirit is a legend that arose in the Heian period (794–1185) about Komyo (701–760), the consort of the Nara period (710–794) emperor Shomu (701–756, reigned 724–749). Shomu is famous for propagating Buddhism in Japan. He ordered the construction of provincial temples, for example, throughout the nation. The provincial temple built for the home province of Yamato became Nara's Todaiji. It houses the Great Buddha, a 16-meter-tall statue of the Vairocana Buddha.

Tradition holds that Komyo was highly influential in nurturing the emperor's religious devotion. She sponsored the construction of facilities to care for the needy, including paupers, invalids, and orphans. In the legend cited here, the empress made a practice of scrubbing residents of those facilities with her own hands. A man who suffered from leprosy appeared while Komyo was engaged in that practice and asked that she scrub him, too. The empress complied, and while she was scrubbing him the man asked her to suck the pus from his ulcerated body. Komyo again complied, whereupon the man revealed himself as the Vajyarana buddha Akshobhya, emanated beams of light from his pores, and ascended into the sky. Akshobhya is a symbol of immovable faith, and his appearance in this legend underlines the profundity of Komyo's religious devotion. We recall here the New Testament episodes where Jesus "cleanses" (heals) a victim of leprosy.

Leprosy also figures in a curious tale recounted in the *Sangoku chori yuraiki* (The origins of the outcasts of three realms), a collection of uncertain provenance. In the tale, the eldest son of the Heian period Emperor Daigo (885–930, reigned 897–930) applied lacquer to his body to simulate leprosy. The prince then took up residence in a district inhabited by outcasts at the foot of Kyoto's Kiyomizuzaka hill. He thereby became something of a patron saint to generations of Japanese who belonged to social groups subject to discrimination.

The belief arose in the Heian period that sites where people gave alms to outcasts, including victims of leprosy, were sacred. People came to believe that Manjushri, the bodhisattva associated with insight and wisdom, appeared at those sites. In the Kamakura period (1185–1333), two Buddhist monks established the practice of cleansing—purifying—the bodies of leprosy victims and other outcasts. The monks were the founder of the Shingon-risshu offshoot of Shingon Buddhism, Eison (1201–1290), and his disciple Ninsho (1217–1303). They regarded their subjects as fleshly manifestations of Manjushri and Akshobhya, and their outreach evinced an accessibility to salvation for all.

Portuguese Jesuits arrived in Japan in the 16th century and carried on the work of tending to leprosy victims as part of their proselytizing. They built leprosaria in Nagasaki and in Osaka, inspired by the biblical teachings encapsulated in the following passage from Matthew:

> When the Son of man shall come in his glory, and all the holy angels with him, then shall he sit upon the throne of his glory: And before him shall be gathered all nations: and he shall separate them one from another, as a shepherd divideth his sheep from the goats: And he shall set the sheep on his right hand, but the goats on the left. Then shall the King say unto them on his right hand, Come, ye blessed of my Father, inherit the kingdom prepared for you from the foundation of the world: For I was an hungred, and ye gave me meat: I was thirsty, and ye gave me drink: I was a stranger, and ye took me in: Naked, and ye clothed me: I was sick, and ye visited me: I was in prison, and ye came unto me. Then shall the righteous answer him, saying, Lord, when saw we thee an hungred, and fed thee? or thirsty, and gave thee drink? When saw we thee a stranger, and took thee in? or naked, and clothed thee? Or when saw we thee sick, or in prison, and came unto thee? And the King shall answer and say unto them, Verily I say unto you, Inasmuch as ye have done it unto one of the least of these my brethren, ye have done it unto me. (Matthew 25:31–40 [KJV])

The Jesuits founded in Nagasaki a chapter of the Misericordia, a charitable organization originated in Rome and that lent aid and solace to condemned convicts and tended to other people in need. In Japan, the Misericordia operated seven facilities to care for such needy individuals as leprosy victims, indigent elderly, and orphans. Its members interpreted and carried out Jesus's teachings in reference to the following seven instructions:

Feed the hungry
Refresh the thirsty
Clothe the naked
Visit the sick
Shelter the homeless
Visit the imprisoned
Bury the dead

Japan's leprosy sufferers needed all the compassion that the Jesuits could provide. They were at the bottom of the social hierarchy. There, they shared with the *eta* untouchables the work of skinning dead animals and disposing of the corpses of execution victims, but they occupied a rung beneath even the *eta* on the social ladder.

A Japanese–Portuguese dictionary published by the Jesuits in Nagasaki in 1603 contains a revealing entry for leather workers. The entry describes a class of leather workers that comprised "individuals who perform the work of removing the skins of dead cattle and other animals and making from them baskets" and who "held the right to oversee persons afflicted with leprosy."

Other historical materials confirm caste-like discrimination far beyond Nagasaki. A 1619 document from the Dewa domain, in Honshu's northwest, verifies that leprosy sufferers were responsible for skinning animals. A 1686 edict by the Sendai domain, Dewa's eastern neighbor, confirms the continuation of discrimination. It specifies that both the *eta* and leprosy sufferers were responsible for disposing of dead horses and cattle and for supplying their skins to the domain and that the *eta* were responsible for overseeing the leprosy sufferers.

The Christian faith exerted a powerful and, in the Edo period, sometimes fateful appeal to sufferers of leprosy. That is evident in chilling records from the Aizu domain, Dewa's neighbor to the south. The shogunate had banned Christianity in 1614, and the Aizu domain executed "numerous lepers" in 1625 for practicing the religion.

Christian missionaries from the West began returning to Japan after the forced reopening of the nation in the 1850s, though an official ban on proselytizing remained in place. Among the missionaries, a Frenchman and two British women established hospitals that cared for victims of leprosy. Germain Léger Testvuide (1849–1891) opened the Koyama Fukusei Hospital in 1889 in the city of Gotemba in what is now Shizuoka Prefecture. Hannah Riddell (1855–1932) opened the Kumamoto Hospital of the Resurrection of Hope in 1895 in the namesake Kyushu city. And Mary Helena Cornwall Legh (1857–1941) opened St. Barnabas' Hospital in 1917 in the city of Kusatsu in what is now Gumma Prefecture. Testvuide's Koyama Fukusei Hospital remains in operation as the oldest leprosy sanatorium in Japan. The government closed Riddell's Kumamoto Hospital of the Resurrection of Hope and Legh's St. Barnabas' Hospital in 1941 and moved the patients to national sanitoriums.

APPENDIX 2

Isolation policy

Japan's policy of isolating sufferers of leprosy from society began at the outset of the 1870s. Russia's Grand Duke Alexei Alexandrovich (1850–1908) was due to pay a goodwill visit in autumn 1872. The Meiji government was embarrassed about the numerous homeless persons who wandered about Tokyo and rounded up about 200 of the homeless and corralled them in quarters out of sight of the Russian visitor. It established a facility on the site of what is now the University of Tokyo's Hongo Campus to house some of the homeless. A lot of the residents were sufferers of leprosy, and the facility therefore included quarters for caring for them in isolation.

The Japanese government conducted the first comprehensive survey of the nationwide prevalence of leprosy in 1900. It carried out the survey through the Home Ministry's Police Affairs Bureau, and the survey turned up 30,359 active cases, which corresponded to 6.43 per 10,000 population. The Home Ministry calculated that 999,300 people in 199,075 households had relatives afflicted by leprosy. Its findings almost certainly undercounted the number of leprosy sufferers on account of the dodgy methodology employed. Even the understated numbers were comparable, however, to the prevalence and potential incidence of the disease in nations less developed than Japan, and they were a shocking revelation for the Japanese.

Adding insult to injury was an incident in 1906. The British ambassador came upon a victim of leprosy who had collapsed in front of the embassy. Appalled, he delivered a protest to Japan's foreign ministry. The ambassador complained that a nation of Japan's standing ought to have facilities to house and care for such unfortunate individuals. A year later, Japan's Diet passed leprosy-prevention legislation.

The leprosy-prevention law was primarily for the purpose of interning homeless sufferers of leprosy in isolation facilities. It required the prefectures to establish and use facilities for that purpose and to disinfect the residences of persons afflicted with leprosy and take other measures for preventing the spread of the disease. The law obliged physicians to notify the authorities whenever they diagnosed a case of leprosy or found leprosy to be the cause of a death. In addition, it obliged the medical authorities to designated specialists to examine individuals diagnosed or suspected of having leprosy.

The toughening and ultimate repeal of the leprosy-prevention law

Japan established a system for operating national leprosaria in 1927 and built the system's first leprosarium three years later on an Okayama Prefecture island in the Seto Naikai inland sea. That facility would become the National Leprosarium Nagashima Aiseien, and its first patients arrived in 1931. The strategy was simple and cold-blooded: Japan would eradicate leprosy by gathering all the members of the populace afflicted by the disease, isolating them from society, preventing them from reproducing, punishing those who tried to escape, and waiting for the internees to die. When the last of the victims had expired, the victory over leprosy would be complete.

The people who administered the anti-leprosy program knew full well that the disease was communicable, not hereditary, and that it was only mildly infectious. Yet they pressed ahead with sadistic abandon. Men underwent forced vasectomies. Women underwent forced abortions when pregnancies occurred despite the leprosaria's thorough measures for segregating the sexes.

The Home Ministry's Central Sanitary Bureau adopted a program in 1930 for eradicating leprosy within 20 years. It estimated that the number of active cases nationwide had declined to about 15,000. The bureau's program provided for interning 5,000 of the afflicted persons in leprosaria already in operation or to be built soon and for expanding the leprosaria capacity within 10 years to accommodate the remaining 10,000 sufferers.

In 1931, the Diet passed leprosy-control legislation that was tougher than the 1907 law in three main respects. One, it empowered the authorities to bar leprosy sufferers from occupations in which they might spread the disease. Two, it restricted the sale or distribution of used bedding and clothing that might be infected with leprosy and prescribed regulations for disinfecting and disposing of such items. And three, it required the authorities to intern leprosy sufferers and suspected leprosy sufferers in national and local government leprosaria and obliged the national and local governments to pay for the internees' upkeep.

The occupational restrictions had the effect of barring sufferers of leprosy from nearly all lines of work. Even more onerous were the toughened internment criteria. Formerly, the leprosy-prevention law had provided only for interning homeless leprosy sufferers. The new law provided for committing all leprosy sufferers, even those living unobtrusively in ordinary households, to the leprosaria. It fed anti-leprosy sentiment, which welled up in the government-sponsored Leprosy-Free Prefectures movement and, notably, in the nationwide lectures and documentary screenings of Leprosy Prevention Day. Those initiatives began in the 1930s and continued, after the interruption of the wartime years, through the 1950s.

Leprosy-prevention legislation passed in 1953 ameliorated some of the more draconian provisions of the 1931 law, but the medically unfounded mandate for isolating leprosy sufferers remained in place. Not until 1996 did the Japanese Diet acknowledge the overpowering weight of scientific evidence and repeal the leprosy-prevention law. Japan's leprosy victims won a historic legal victory in 2001 with a ruling by the Kumamoto district court. The court ruled in favor of 127 plaintiffs who had argued that their forced internment had been unconstitutional, and the court's judgment took hold when Prime Minister Junichiro Koizumi declined to contest the ruling. Japan's leprosy sufferers were free at last.

APPENDIX 3

RESOLUTION AND PRINCIPLES AND GUIDELINES ADOPTED UNANIMOUSLY BY THE UN GENERAL ASSEMBLY ON DECEMBER 21, 2010

The General Assembly,

Recalling the provisions of the Universal Declaration of Human Rights, including article 1, which states that all human beings are born free and equal in dignity and rights, and that they are endowed with reason and conscience and should act towards one another in a spirit of brotherhood,

Recalling also relevant Human Rights Council resolutions 8/13 of 18 June 2008, 12/7 of 1 October 2009 and 15/10 of 30 September 2010,

Reaffirming that persons affected by leprosy and their family members should be treated as individuals with dignity and are entitled to all human rights and fundamental freedoms under customary international law, relevant conventions and national constitutions and laws,

1. Welcomes the work of the Human Rights Council and takes note with appreciation of the work of Human Rights Council Advisory Committee on the elimination of discrimination against persons affected by leprosy and their family members;

2. Takes note with appreciation of the Principles and Guidelines for the elimination of discrimination against persons affected by leprosy and their family members;

3. Encourages Governments, relevant United Nations bodies, specialized agencies, funds and programmes, other intergovernmental organizations and national human rights institutions to give due consideration to the Principles and Guidelines in the formulation and implementation of their policies and measures concerning persons affected by leprosy and their family members;

4. Encourages all relevant actors in society, including hospitals, schools, universities, religious groups and organizations, business enterprises,

newspapers, broadcasting networks and other non-governmental organizations, to give due consideration, as appropriate, to the Principles and Guidelines, in the course of their activities.

Principles and Guidelines

I. Principles

1. Persons affected by leprosy and their family members should be treated as people with dignity and are entitled, on an equal basis with others, to all the human rights and fundamental freedoms proclaimed in the Universal Declaration of Human Rights, as well as in other relevant international human rights instruments to which their respective States are parties, including the International Covenant on Economic, Social and Cultural Rights, the International Covenant on Civil and Political Rights, and the Convention on the Rights of Persons with Disabilities.
2. Persons affected by leprosy and their family members should not be discriminated against on the grounds of having or having had leprosy.
3. Persons affected by leprosy and their family members should have the same rights as everyone else with respect to marriage, family and parenthood. To this end:
   (a) No one should be denied the right to marry on the grounds of leprosy;
   (b) Leprosy should not constitute a ground for divorce;
   (c) A child should not be separated from his or her parents on the grounds of leprosy.
4. Persons affected by leprosy and their family members should have the same rights as everyone else in relation to full citizenship and obtaining identity documents.
5. Persons affected by leprosy and their family members should have the right to serve the public, on an equal basis with others, including the right to stand for elections and to hold office at all levels of government.
6. Persons affected by leprosy and their family members should have the right to work in an environment that is inclusive and to be treated on an equal basis with others in all policies and processes related to recruitment, hiring, promotion, salary, continuance of employment and career advancement.
7. Persons affected by leprosy and their family members should not be denied admission to or be expelled from schools or training programmes on the grounds of leprosy.

8. Persons affected by leprosy and their family members are entitled to develop their human potential to the fullest extent, and to fully realize their dignity and self-worth. Persons affected by leprosy and their family members who have been empowered and who have had the opportunity to develop their abilities can be powerful agents of social change.

9. Persons affected by leprosy and their family members have the right to be, and should be, actively involved in decision-making processes regarding policies and programmes that directly concern their lives.

II. Guidelines

1. General

1.1 States should promote, protect and ensure the full realization of all human rights and fundamental freedoms for all persons affected by leprosy and their family members without discrimination on the grounds of leprosy. To this end, States should:

(a) Take all appropriate legislative, administrative and other measures to modify, repeal or abolish existing laws, regulations, policies, customs and practices that discriminate directly or indirectly against persons affected by leprosy and their family members, or that forcefully or compulsorily segregate and isolate persons on the grounds of leprosy in the context of such discrimination;

(b) Ensure that all authorities and institutions take measures to eliminate discrimination on the grounds of leprosy by any person, organization or private enterprise.

1.2 States should take all appropriate measures to achieve for persons affected by leprosy and their family members the full realization of all the rights enshrined in the Universal Declaration of Human Rights and the international human rights instruments to which they are party, including the International Covenant on Economic, Social and Cultural Rights, the International Covenant on Civil and Political Rights and the Convention on the Rights of Persons with Disabilities.

1.3 In the development and implementation of legislation and policies and in other decision-making processes concerning issues relating to persons affected by leprosy and their family members, States should consult closely with and actively involve persons affected by leprosy and their family members, individually or through their respective local and national organizations.

2. Equality and non-discrimination

2.1   States should recognize that all persons are equal before and under the law and are entitled, without any discrimination, to the equal protection and equal benefit of the law.

2.2   States should prohibit all discrimination on the grounds of a person having or having had leprosy, and should guarantee equal and effective legal protection to persons affected by leprosy and their family members.

2.3   Specific measures which are necessary to achieve de facto equality of persons affected by leprosy and their family members shall not be considered as discrimination.

3. Women, children and other vulnerable groups

3.1   In many societies, leprosy has a significantly adverse impact on women, children and other vulnerable groups. States should therefore pay special attention to the promotion and protection of the human rights of women, children and members of other vulnerable groups who have or have had leprosy, as well as their family members.

3.2   States should promote the full development, advancement and empowerment of women, children and members of other vulnerable groups who have or have had leprosy, as well as their family members.

4. Home and family

States should, where possible, support the reunification of families separated in the past as a result of policies and practices relating to persons diagnosed with leprosy.

5. Living in the community and housing

5.1   States should promote the enjoyment of the same rights for persons affected by leprosy and their family members as for everyone else, allowing their full inclusion and participation in the community.

5.2   States should identify persons affected by leprosy and their family members living in isolation or segregated from their community because of their disease, and should give them social support.

5.3   States should enable persons affected by leprosy and their family members to choose their place of residence and should ensure that they are not obliged to accept a particular living arrangement because of their disease.

5.4   States should allow any persons affected by leprosy and their family members who were once forcibly isolated by State policies in effect at the time to continue to live in the leprosariums and hospitals that have become their homes, if they so desire. In the event that relocation is unavoidable, the residents of these places should be active participants in decisions concerning their future. States should, however, improve living conditions in those leprosariums and hospitals. With due regard to the wishes of the persons affected by leprosy and their family members, and with their full participation, States should also design, promote and implement plans for the gradual integration of the residents of such places in the community and for the gradual phasing out of such leprosariums and hospitals.

6. Participation in political life

States should ensure that persons affected by leprosy, and their family members, enjoy voting rights, the right to stand for election and the right to hold public office at all levels of government, on an equal basis with others. Voting procedures must be accessible, easy to use and adapted to accommodate any individuals physically affected by leprosy.

7. Occupation

States should encourage and support opportunities for self-employment, the formation of cooperatives and vocational training for persons affected by leprosy and their family members, as well as their employment in regular labour markets.

8. Education

States should promote equal access to education for persons affected by leprosy and their family members.

9. Discriminatory language

States should remove discriminatory language, including the derogatory use of the term "leper" or its equivalent in any language or dialect, from governmental publications and should revise expeditiously, where possible, existing publications containing such language.

10. Participation in public, cultural and recreational activities

10.1 States should promote the equal enjoyment of the rights and freedoms of persons affected by leprosy and their family members, as enshrined in the Universal Declaration of Human Rights and the international human rights instruments to which they are party, including the International

Covenant on Economic, Social and Cultural Rights, the International Covenant on Civil and Political Rights and the Convention on the Rights of Persons with Disabilities.

10.2 States should promote access on an equal basis with others to public places, including hotels, restaurants and buses, trains and other forms of public transport for persons affected by leprosy and their family members.

10.3 States should promote access on an equal basis with others to cultural and recreational facilities for persons affected by leprosy and their family members.

10.4 States should promote access on an equal basis with others to places of worship for persons affected by leprosy and their family members.

11. Health care

11.1 States should provide persons affected by leprosy at least with the same range, quality and standard of free or affordable health care as that provided for persons with other diseases. In addition, States should provide for early detection programmes and ensure prompt treatment of leprosy, including treatment for any reactions and nerve damage that may occur, in order to prevent the development of stigmatic consequences.

11.2 States should include psychological and social counselling as standard care offered to persons affected by leprosy who are undergoing diagnosis and treatment, and as needed after the completion of treatment.

11.3 States should ensure that persons affected by leprosy have access to free medication for leprosy, as well as appropriate health care.

12. Standard of living

12.1 States should recognize the right of persons affected by leprosy and their family members to an adequate standard of living, and should take appropriate steps to safeguard and promote that right, without discrimination on the grounds of leprosy, with regard to food, clothing, housing, drinking water, sewage systems and other living conditions. States should:

(a) Promote collaborative programmes involving the Government, civil society and private institutions to raise funds and develop programmes to improve the standard of living;

(b) Provide or ensure the provision of education to children whose families are living in poverty by means of scholarships and other programmes sponsored by the Government and/or civil society;

(c) Ensure that persons living in poverty have access to vocational training programmes, microcredit and other means to improve their standard of living.

12.2 States should promote the realization of this right through financial measures, such as the following:

(a) Persons affected by leprosy and their family members who are not able to work because of their age, illness or disability should be provided with a government pension;

(b) Persons affected by leprosy and their family members who are living in poverty should be provided with financial assistance for housing and health care.

13. Awareness-raising

States, working with human rights institutions, non-governmental organizations, civil society and the media, should formulate policies and plans of action to raise awareness throughout society and to foster respect for the rights and dignity of persons affected by leprosy and their family members. These policies and plans of action may include the following goals:

(a) To provide information about leprosy at all levels of the education system, beginning with early childhood education affirming, inter alia, that leprosy is curable and should not be used as grounds for discrimination against persons who have or have had leprosy and their families;

(b) To promote the production and dissemination of "know your rights" material to give to all persons recently diagnosed with leprosy;

(c) To encourage the media to portray persons affected by leprosy and their family members with dignified images and terminology;

(d) To recognize the skills, merits and abilities of persons affected by leprosy and their contribution to society and, where possible, to support exhibitions of their artistic, cultural and scientific talents;

(e) To encourage creative persons, including artists, poets, musicians and writers, particularly those who have personally faced the challenges of leprosy, to make a contribution to awareness-raising through their specific talents;

(f) To provide information to social leaders, including religious leaders, on how addressing leprosy in their teachings or written materials may contribute to the elimination of discrimination against persons affected by the disease and their family members;

(g) To encourage higher education institutions, including medical schools and nursing schools, to include information about leprosy in their curricula, and to develop and implement a "train the trainer" programme and targeted educational materials;

(h) To promote implementation of the World Programme for Human Rights Education and to incorporate the human rights of persons affected by leprosy and their family members into the national human rights education programme of each State;

(i) To identify ways to recognize, honour and learn from the lives of individuals forcibly isolated by their Governments for having been diagnosed with leprosy, including oral history programmes, museums, monuments and publications;

(j) To support grass-roots awareness efforts to reach communities without access to traditional media.

14. Development, implementation and follow-up to States' activities

14.1 States should consider creating or designating a committee to address activities relating to the human rights of persons affected by leprosy and their family members. The committee should ideally include individuals affected by leprosy and their family members, representatives of organizations of persons affected by leprosy, human rights experts, representatives from the human rights field and related fields, and representatives of government.

14.2 States are encouraged to include in their State party reports to the relevant treaty bodies the policies and measures that they have adopted and/or implemented with regard to the elimination of discrimination against persons affected by leprosy and their family members.

APPENDIX 4

INTERNATIONAL SYMPOSIUM
TOWARDS HOLISTIC CARE FOR PEOPLE WITH HANSEN'S DISEASE, RESPECTFUL OF THEIR DIGNITY (VATICAN CITY, 9–10 JUNE 2016)

Conclusions and Recommendations

The International Symposium on the topic, "Towards Holistic Care for People with Hansen's Disease, Respectful of Their Dignity," was jointly organized for June 9 to 10, 2016, at the Vatican City by the Pontifical Council for Health Care Workers, the Good Samaritan Foundation and the Nippon Foundation in cooperation with the Fondation Raoul Follereau, the Sovereign Order of Malta and the Sasakawa Memorial Health Foundation. These Conclusions and Recommendations were presented at the end of the two-day symposium and were approved in principle by the organizers and the participants who were present.

Note

While the terms "Hansen's disease" and "leprosy" are used interchangeably in this document, in some countries the preferred term is Hansen's disease.

Conclusions

1. Every new case of Hansen's disease is one case too many.

It has been observed that new cases of Hansen's disease are on the decrease and we should be very happy about this. But this decrease, which is in itself positive, could have resulted from a decline in case-finding activities and reduced community awareness. The increase in the rate of disabilities in new cases detected seems to support this explanation. Therefore, it is essential to aim at early detection. This applies to all new cases, but particularly to child cases. The WHO's Global Leprosy Strategy 2016-2020 is moving in this direction. A second cause for concern comes from the substantial risk of partly losing the expertise that has been accumulated over recent decades by leprosy experts, medical doctors and health workers in relation to Hansen's disease. Grants for study and training may be needed for service providers and caretakers including persons affected by the disease. Here, the principle, "Nothing about us without us" should be respected, and this is an important way of fighting against the stigma that is associated with Hansen's disease. A number of valuable recommendations in the presentations concerned methods to improve early diagnosis and promote the social integration of persons affected by leprosy. Public and private institutions should work in close cooperation with health authorities in each country to provide medical and health personnel with basic education about leprosy in order to strengthen leprosy programs within the framework of general health services. Efforts should be made to reintegrate communities of persons affected by leprosy into society. The message that leprosy is curable and can be treated while the patient continues to live at home should be emphasized.

2. Every case of stigma and social exclusion is one case too many.

Stigma is often associated with a religious vision of life and it would be advisable to revise this belief. In reality, stigma has been linked from the earliest times with fear of a disease that cannot be defeated. Biblical texts of the Old Testament themselves record a practice of exclusion that was present in Egyptian, Assyrian-Babylonian and Canaanite cultures during the second millennium before Christ. The same fear is to be found in non-Christian and non-religious contexts. The teaching of Christ in the New Testament, first of all, breaks, with great clarity, the connection between illness and sin (John 9:2-3). Secondly, Jesus Christ touches people with leprosy, enters into contact with a sick person without any fear of contagion or impurity, and heals and reintegrates people into the community. Even more, he himself accepts being treated as if he had leprosy. The example of Christ has often not been followed—this neglect enables us to understand that it is easier to eliminate the disease at a medical level than the social prejudice that surrounds it. In this sense, it is absolutely necessary that we place the human being at the centre of all medical activity, rather than, as is often the case, placing the disease at the centre of attention.

It is the teaching of Christ which has led Christians, especially over the last two centuries, to develop a high level of care and treatment for people with Hansen's disease. This took place even before pharmacological therapies were available, when care involved accepting and rescuing people and ending their state of abandonment. There is no need to recall here the giants of charity who were dedicated to this service. Today, as well, the Catholic Church remains strongly committed in almost all countries where the disease is found, to providing medical and humanistic care. Here a pathway opens up of cooperation with religious communities of other faiths and with all men and women of good will.

It is the shared opinion of experts who work in the field of Hansen's disease that the elimination of the stigma attached to leprosy requires an important work of education that must involve all social groups and in particular religious communities because they promote respect for human dignity throughout the world.

3. Every law that discriminates against people affected by Hansen's disease is one law too many.

Following intensive work, the General Assembly of the United Nations in December 2010 adopted a resolution on elimination of discrimination against persons affected by leprosy and their family members, accompanied by "Principles and Guidelines". The resolution and "Principles and Guidelines" constitute a milestone in the upholding of the human rights of persons affected by Hansen's disease. One must take into account that for every person with the disease, his or her family members and even relatives may also be ostracized due to the stigma attached to leprosy, resulting in a serious violation of fundamental human rights. An enormous amount of work still has to be done by governments and social and religious institutions to ensure that these "Principles and Guidelines" are fully implemented.

Unfortunately, various forms of discrimination continue to exist in many parts of the world which bear upon all spheres of life: schools, workplaces, social groups, public places, religious centres, restaurants, hotels, trains and other means of transport. Especially grave are the violations of the rights of persons affected by leprosy in the field of education, work, and marriage. The necessity to repeal discriminatory laws that impede fundamental human rights is very urgent and can no longer be postponed.

Implementation of the "Principles and Guidelines" requires constant work involving the sensitization of governments and societies. To this end, in 2012 the Nippon Foundation created a working group (the International Working Group, hereafter IWG), which had the aim of assisting the process of implementation of the "Principles and Guidelines". The IWG prepared a "Suggested Framework for National Plans of Action" for States to use in their own domestic contexts. The IWG came to the conclusion that the "Principles and Guidelines" were more likely to be effective if States were called upon to undertake specific ways of implementing them, which could then be brought to the attention of various governmental offices and communicated to relevant UN bodies, specialized agencies, funds and programmes, other intergovernmental organizations and national human rights institutions. To this end, the IWG recommended the institution of a follow-up mechanism at an international level which would have the mandate to follow up the actions of States and other stakeholders, drawing upon the experience of Special Rapporteurs on various topics of human rights appointed by the United Nations Human Rights Council, or committees of experts which monitor the implementation of international human rights treaties and conventions. This follow-up work must not be neglected, otherwise there will be no perception of progress or steps back. Accordingly, in the Resolution adopted by the UN Human Rights Council on 2 July 2015, the UN Human Rights Council Advisory Committee is requested to submit a report containing practical suggestions for the wider dissemination and more effective implementation of the 'Principles and Guidelines' at the 35th session of the United Nations Human Rights Council in June 2017.

The IWG has observed, in particular, the need for civil society and religious communities to use dignified terminology when speaking about Hansen's disease. It has been observed that the old perceptions of leprosy continue to be reinforced by inappropriate language. The offensive term 'leper' as a description of someone with leprosy evokes a marginalized person, a sinner, or a person who is rejected by other people for moral or social reasons. This terminology contributes to discrimination against persons affected by leprosy and even discourages those who need treatment from seeking help. The IWG has thus invited religious leaders and their communities to reflect upon the best ways of expressing themselves in language that is able to transmit respect for persons affected by leprosy. Awareness-raising activities at the global level should make full use of new media to inform people about advances in treatment of leprosy and the fact that people who are under treatment or have completed treatment are not infectious. It is important that this information is available even in countries where leprosy is not an issue, in order to eliminate the myths surrounding this disease.

Final Recommendations

Two Introductory Points

1. Persons affected by Hansen's disease must be seen as the main actors in the fight against this disease and the discrimination it causes. This involvement

is a powerful instrument for the recognition of their equal dignity and rights for social inclusion, and for the breaking of the stigma attached to them. This point applies to all of the recommendations listed below.

2. The use of discriminatory language that reinforces stigma must cease, in particular, use of the term 'leper' and its equivalent in other languages. This term is offensive for the reasons stated above and also because it defines a person by his or her illness. Use of the term "leprosy" in a metaphorical sense should be avoided.

Five Recommendations

1. Given their important role in their respective communities of believers, the leaders of all religions—and this is an important and urgent matter— should, in their teachings, writings and speeches, contribute to the elimination of discrimination against persons affected by leprosy by spreading awareness that leprosy is curable and stressing that there is no reason to discriminate against anyone affected by leprosy or members of their families.

2. States and governments should be encouraged to make great efforts to implement the "Principles and Guidelines" accompanying the resolution adopted by the General Assembly of the United Nations in 2010 on elimination of discrimination against persons affected by leprosy and their family members. These "Principles and Guidelines" must be fully implemented, otherwise they will remain just empty proclamations.

3. There should be a modification or abolition of all laws and regulations that discriminate against persons affected by leprosy. Policies relating to family, work, schools, or any other areas which directly or indirectly discriminate against persons affected by leprosy must also be changed, recognizing that no one must be discriminated against because of the fact that he or she has, or once had, leprosy.

4. There is a need for further scientific research to develop new medical tools to prevent and treat leprosy and its complications, and to achieve better diagnostic methods.

5. In order to achieve a world free of leprosy and the discrimination it causes, the efforts of all the Churches, religious communities, international organizations, governments, major foundations, NGOs, and associations of persons affected by leprosy which have hitherto contributed to the fight against this disease should be unified and joint plans of cooperation should be developed.

APPENDIX 5

YOHEI SASAKAWA AND THE FIGHT AGAINST LEPROSY OVER THE YEARS

		Yohei Sasakawa or Nippon Foundation	*Other leprosy-related events*
1965	September	Develops interest in fighting leprosy after accompanying father, Ryoichi, on visit to leprosarium in Republic of Korea	
1968	October		9th International Leprosy Congress, London
1973	August		10th International Leprosy Congress, Bergen, Norway
1974	May	Japan Foundation for Shipbuilding Advancement establishes Sasakawa Memorial Health Foundation and concurrently begins extending financial assistance to WHO	
1978	November		11th International Leprosy Congress, Mexico City
1981	January	Becomes chairman of Tokyo Motorboat Racing Association	

	February	Becomes vice-chairman of Japan Motorboat Racing Association	
	February	Becomes trustee of Japan Shipbuilding Industry Foundation	
			WHO study group recommends multidrug therapy as cure for leprosy
1983	May	Accompanies Ryoichi to Vatican for audience with Pope John Paul II. Begins devoting energy wholeheartedly to fight against leprosy	
1984	February		12th International Leprosy Congress, New Delhi
1987	December	Ryoichi receives world's first leprosy-prevention vaccination at WHO headquarters	
1988	March	Becomes acting president of Japan Shipbuilding Industry Foundation	
	September		13th International Leprosy Congress, The Hague
1989	May	Becomes president of Japan Shipbuilding Industry Foundation	
1991	May		44th World Health Assembly adopts resolution that calls for

			eliminating leprosy as public health problem by 2000
1993	August		14th International Leprosy Congress, Orlando
1994		Announces at leprosy-control conference in Hanoi that Japan Shipbuilding Industry Foundation will donate $50 million to WHO to fund free distribution of multidrug therapy for five years, starting in 1995	
1995	July	Ryoichi dies	
1996	January	Japan Shipbuilding Industry Foundation adopts "Nippon Foundation" as informal name	
	April		Japanese Diet repeals leprosy-prevention law
1997			Sponsors photographic exhibition at UN headquarters that introduces persons affected by leprosy and their quest for dignity
1998	September		15th International Leprosy Congress, Beijing
1999		Participates in launching Global Alliance for the Elimination of Leprosy	WHO adopts target of bringing leprosy under control in all nations by end of 2005

2001	January		Global Alliance for the Elimination of Leprosy holds first meeting in New Delhi and issues call for bringing leprosy under control in all nations by 2005
	May	Named Special Ambassador for Global Alliance for the Elimination of Leprosy	
	May	Becomes Special Ambassador for the Global Alliance for the Elimination of Leprosy (becomes WHO Goodwill Ambassador for Leprosy Elimination in 2004)	Kumamoto district court rules in favor of former leprosy patients who charged that treatment under leprosy-prevention law was unconstitutional. Ruling takes hold when government declines to appeal
	October	Delivers keynote address on human rights dimension of leprosy at Forum 2000 international conference in Prague	
2002	August		16th International Leprosy Congress, Salvador, Brazil
	October	Has audience with Pope John Paul II at Vatican and reports on status of measures for bringing leprosy under control	
2003	July	Makes first visit to Office of the United Nations High Commissioner for Human Rights and begins pressing	

		for addressing leprosy as human rights issue	
2004	January		African Leprosy Congress, Johannesburg
	January		Leprosy-elimination conference, Mumbai
	March	Delivers speech on subject of leprosy and human rights at regular session of UN Commission on Human Rights	
	August		UN Sub-Commission on the Promotion and Protection of Human Rights resolves to conduct leprosy study from human rights perspective
2005	May		UN Sub-Commission on the Promotion and Protection of Human Rights adopts resolution that calls for ending discrimination against persons affected by leprosy
	July	Becomes chairman of Japan Shipbuilding Industry Foundation	
	August		UN Sub-Commission on the Promotion and Protection of Human Rights adopts resolution that calls for ending discrimination against

			leprosy patients and former patients and their family members
	December	Participates in New Delhi gathering for establishing National Forum as network of about 700 Indian leprosy colonies and becomes inaugural chairman	
2006	January	Launches Global Appeal to End Stigma and Discrimination against Persons Affected by Leprosy in New Delhi	
	January		Indian government announces nation's attainment of WHO benchmark for leprosy control
	August		UN Sub-Commission on the Promotion and Protection of Human Rights adopts resolution that calls for continued deliberations by UN Human Rights Council on elimination of leprosy-related discrimination
	November	Launches Sasakawa-India Leprosy Foundation	
2007	September	Named Japanese government's Goodwill Ambassador for the Human Rights of Persons Affected by Leprosy	

2008	January		17th International Leprosy Congress, Hyderabad
	June	Writes letter to Chinese organizing committee for 2008 Beijing Olympic Games to protest visa restrictions on visitors afflicted by leprosy (Chinese government subsequently lifts restrictions)	
2010	September		Resolution on "Elimination of discrimination against persons affected by leprosy and their family members" and accompanying set of principles and guidelines for fulfilling resolution receive unanimous approval by members of UN Human Rights Council
	December		Above resolution and principles and guidelines receive unanimous approval by 192 delegates at UN General Assembly
2011	April	Japan Shipbuilding Industry Foundation changes name to Nippon Foundation (unofficial name since 1996)	

2012	January	Writes letter to Sony Pictures to protest offensive portrayal of leprosy in animated feature film. Sony Pictures subsequently amends offensive portion of film	
	August	Has audience with Dalai Lama in Dharamsala, India. Secures promise from Dalai Lama to visit leprosy colony in New Delhi (fulfilled in August 2014)	
2013	June	Writes letter to Pope Francis to protest pontiff's use of language discriminatory to victims of leprosy	
	September		18th International Leprosy Congress, Brussels
2016	February		Fifty-nine former leprosy patients (number increases to 509 in March) file suit against national government in Kumamoto district court that seeks damages of ¥5 million per person and formal apology
	June	Nippon Foundation cosponsors leprosy symposium with Vatican	

Awards (partial listing)

Health and Human Rights Award, International Council of Nurses (2017); Rule of Law Award, International Bar Association (2014); International Gandhi Award, Gandhi Memorial Leprosy Foundation (2007); Millennium Gandhi Award, International Leprosy Union (2001); Health-for-All Gold Medal, WHO (1998)

Honorary degrees

University of Minnesota (2017); Sofia University (2016); University of York (2013); University of Malaya (2012); Hawassa University, Ethiopia (2012); Russian Academy of Natural Science (2010); Yunnan University (2009); University for Peace, Costa Rica (2008); Dalian University of Foreign Languages (2008); University of Cambodia (2007); Guizhou University (2007); Rochester Institute of Technology, United States (2007); Dalian Maritime University (2006); Jadavpur University, India (2005); Shanghai Maritime University (2004); World Maritime University, Sweden (2004); Heilongjiang University (2004); Harbin Medical University (2004); China Medical University (2003); Academy of Management, Mongolia (2003); University of Bucharest (2000); University of Cape Coast, Ghana (2000); Yanbian University (2000)

INDEX